Good Morning, Blake

Growing Up Autistic and Being Okay

Blake "Crash" Priddle

Memories are funny things—some are crystal clear, some are fuzzy. We each have our own recollection of events. This book is a compilation of our memories. I have represented people and my life's events as best as I can remember them. Nothing I write is meant to hurt anyone. A few names have been changed for privacy. A few events occurred in different chronological order than presented but are factual.

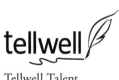

Tellwell Talent
www.tellwell.ca

ISBN
978-0-2288-5969-7 (Hardcover)
978-0-2288-5967-3 (Paperback)
978-0-2288-5968-0 (eBook)

Praise for *Good Morning, Blake*

"Wow. This book is a must read. It's an eye-opening, honest exploration of a beautiful life. If you are lucky enough to love someone on the spectrum, do yourself (and them) a favour and read this book. Never a dull moment, the collaborative style in which Blake writes is both informative and riveting, and he illuminates so many points of view that readers will feel immersed in the story while also learning amazing insights and information. Somewhere between a scrapbook and a personal diary, with pictures, thoughts from parents and caregivers, this book offers insight and new ways to think and love and live. We are excited for a chance to learn about what it feels like to be Blake, and through this we are able to connect more deeply, and that is really the most important part of life...so thank you Blake for giving us all an opportunity to see the world through your eyes. We look forward to the sequel and the next chapter in your life!

Taes and Nick (Splash'N Boots) www.splashnboots.com

This book is just wonderful! I was so taken with everything that was written. Blake shows the raw and most sincere feelings of autism. He tells it as it is while teaching those who are reading it. As I read each chapter, I was immediately thinking of people who I would send this book to for them to read. I could visualize many of the children and young adults in our community as I read the stories and his challenges. They would certainly learn a lot from reading this book.

Joan Chaisson, co-founder of Autism Involves Me (AIM), and Canada's Most Autism-Friendly Town, Port aux Basques, Newfoundland and Labrador

Blake's story shows us how essential acceptance and community support is to help our youth with autism thrive as adults. A strong foundation is vital to help people develop confidence, resilience and competence in not only their chosen field but also in their adult life in general. Blake has been very fortunate to be surrounded by people who see and nurture his abilities and who have inspired him to hold the door open for those coming behind him. It is great to have someone like him in a community acting as a role model for children with autism.

Melanie Wallcraft Young, mom of autistic child and founder of The Pas and Area Autism Group, Manitoba

We have much to learn about the demands of living with a lifelong condition. Blake presents how difficult this is and the commitment and courage required. I have been diagnosed with Parkinson's disease, which is different but we have commonalities. I tell people that, yes, I am facing life with a chronic condition but while it will always accompany me in my life journey, I work hard so that I stay in the driver's seat. Blake had to master this lesson much earlier in life than most and continue to work at it every day. Sharing his story is valuable to many. I like the title. It states up front—I may have a condition but I am okay (I am still in the driver's seat...).

Louise Picard, nursing researcher and advocate. Recipient of an honorary doctorate from Laurentian University for dedication to improving her community

As a mother of special needs children, I understand the stigma attached with illness, no matter what it is. Perhaps those experiences led me to not be taken aback by Blake's autism but to embrace it. Blake has always impressed me; he has a big heart and tries so hard to do the best job he can. He is a positive role model for anyone on the spectrum... his commercials, radio work, journalism, as well as his activism and volunteering are what makes Blake! Sharing those positives in his book will continue to change people's views.

Rosalind "Roz" Russell, media personality

Blake's memory of his early years is remarkable. I love the format—the chronological order. The reader learns so much and grows along with Blake. A heavy subject endearingly told that makes us laugh and cry and feel many emotions in between. Also highlights the importance of journaling—love that! Congratulations to Blake and his huge village—especially mayors Jo and Ted.

Marg Turner, former journalist

Dedicated to...

Everyone who cares, lives with or
includes autism in their lives.

*"Principles focusing on equality and fairness,
those are principles that we can't let go of."*

Niki Ashton
Member of Parliament, Churchill-Keewatinook Aski, Manitoba

Table of Contents

**Chapter 3. My Teen Years: Surviving
and Thriving in High School**

Foreword

(as told by my mom)

Three words changed my life.

"Good morning, Blake," I said as I entered my toddler's room one sunny fall morning. There he was, standing in his crib, beaming that most lovable grin and jumping up and down on his tippy toes, excited to see me, his mom.

"Good morning, Blake," he squealed back to me.

I froze.

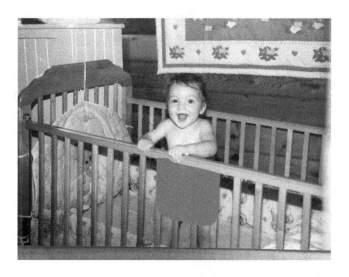

Good morning, Blake!

Armed with a master's degree in child development and being an aunt and friend to many young kids, I knew this was not the "right" response for an eighteen-month-old. He should have said, "Up mommy, I want up, hi mommy..." But no, instead he echoed back what he heard me say. I knew in that instant, as my heart pounded and my gut wretched, that my world was now orbiting a completely different path than I had ever imagined.

Fast forward a quarter century and I can now say that those were the best three words I have ever heard. I have not always felt like this—it has taken me years to figure out this parenting thing and to really step back (and forward) to understand our world and how those who are "disabled" and "different" should be treated. As I look back, I believe Nelson Mandela's words capture how I feel about this journey Blake writes about. Mandela said, "There can be no keener revelation of a society's soul than the way in which it treats its children," and, "Difficulties break some men, but make others."

This book is about growing up autistic and being okay. It is Blake's memoir recounted by Blake and others. It has always been his goal to write about his life. He thought that it would be insightful to have his mom's journal format perspective parallel some of his stories.

What makes this book unique is that Blake reached out, interviewed and received stories from over fifty peers, family members, friends, teachers and work colleagues. Some have known him all his life, others for short periods in his development. Blake told them not to worry about embarrassing or insulting him or feeling bad writing things that might be hard, awkward, sad or odd. Contributors also shared helpful tips or strategies to pass on to others who have autism or who share their lives with others who do. This exceptional feature of his book demonstrates that "it takes a village to raise a kid."

Blake has written a book that is a "feel good," positive book, but he has not sugar-coated things. It's not inspiration porn. After all, life is full of ups and downs, and that is okay. This isn't a *Dummies' Guide to Autism*, the definitive evidence-based treatment manual or a perfectly politically correct perspective on life (some terms and stories may not use the latest PC words—sorry). It also isn't a trajectory for all folks on the autism spectrum. It is simply Blake's story, told by Blake.

Enjoy his journey.

Jo Beyers (Blake's Mom)

Introduction

One word: *Autistic.*

It evokes emotions, stereotypes, hopes, dreams, worries and wonders.

Parents and autistic self-advocates, like myself, Blake "Crash" Priddle (I'll explain the "Crash" later on), turn to innumerable sources of information to gain a handle on this disability, this other-worldly way of being and viewing the world. My parents and I have gleaned a lot of insight from one such source—Dr. Temple Grandin. While not representative of all folks on the autism spectrum, Dr. Grandin is an extraordinary role model. She broke from the mould of being institutionalized in the 1950s. Her mother did everything in her power to shape her daughter's development and the environments she lived in. Today, Dr. Grandin is an expert in livestock facility design and an international lecturer on autism.

Wise Words from Dr. Temple Grandin

In a 2016 interview, Dr. Grandin shared her views on what it takes for autistic individuals to reach their full potential. Here's an excerpt:

Interviewer: I'd like to chat with you about what tips you'd give to help autistic people reach their full potential. What would you tell the parents to do?

Temple Grandin: I have to tell parents, depending on the age of their kid, if you have a three-year-old who's not talking, you need to get him into a really good early intervention program. I recommend they start doing jobs when they're in middle school—paper route, walking dogs. Getting job experience before they graduate from high school and college is a really good idea.

Interviewer: Eighty-five percent of adults with autism are either unemployed or under-employed. What will it take to change this problem so that more folks on the spectrum have meaningful paid work?

Temple Grandin: Well, the way I got paid work was being really good at what I do. And selling to people based on the portfolio of my work designing cattle facilities, writing articles for cattle magazines. That's how I started. Get really good at a skill other people want. I would take my drawings out and show them, and they'd go, "Oh, you did that?" And then I would get a job at another feed yard to design a facility. Get good at something because you're not going to do very well in the job interview[1].

Interviewer: What workplace accommodations have helped you succeed?

Temple Grandin: Well, fortunately there were some good people in the cattle industry that helped me. The movie (*Temple Grandin,* 2010) showed people that were bad and good to me. The boss needs to just help and coach the person on some of the social mistakes, and they can't be vague.

Surprise! It's Me!

You may be wondering who conducted this interview with one of the most well-known people with autism. Well, it was me, Blake "Crash" Priddle. You will see how significant this is as you read my story and many others'.

I decided to share the story of my life for a couple of reasons. With 85% of my autistic peers not meaningfully employed, what facilitators occurred in my life to break from this dismal statistic and find and keep a job? I'd like to give people with autism spectrum disorder (ASD) and their families hope—to inspire people like me to do whatever they dream of while at the same time giving parents a light at the end of a sometimes dark tunnel.

It was difficult for me to make friends as a kid, and even now it is still a challenge. I've joined community activities like theatre, the

---

[1]   Despite possessing essential job skills, differences in the way that autistic people understand and respond to others in social situations mean they are often disadvantaged in job interviews.

Lion's Club, darts, fishing derbies and the local autism chapter to meet like-minded people. I spend my spare time hunting, fishing and hiking in the bush. When it's forty below you can find me writing novellas, painting landscape scenes or watching funny shows on my iPad.

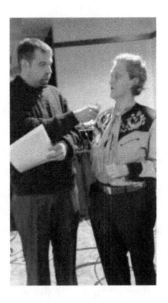

Me interviewing Temple Grandin, 2016, Sault Ste. Marie, Ontario *(courtesy D. Lendrum)*

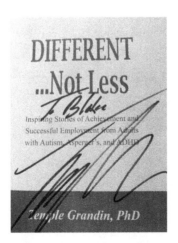

Book by Temple Grandin, signed to me

Today I am a news reporter and radio personality. This is the story of my life growing up with autism. I wasn't really verbal until I was about five, and when I did talk, I had echolalia[2] and difficulty understanding what people were saying. Fast forward twenty plus years and here I am—making a living TALKING on the radio! How did this come about?

Many would say that a person with autism could never work in journalism because it's a very social and fast-paced field—skills autistics struggle with. It is safe to say I proved a lot of people wrong. Working in media helps me come out of my shell. I continue to need occasional support. I live in a remote northern part of Canada, in Manitoba. I would still be living in my parents' basement[3] if it wasn't for all the amazing support of my teachers, college profs, family, therapists, friends and mentors. They never gave up on me, and they all found ways to make sure I would be successful—by believing in me.

I'm not going to lie to you—there have been and continue to be many ups and downs in my journey to becoming a successful radio guy. Autism usually comes with other issues—in my case I struggle from time to time with obsessive-compulsive disorder (OCD), anxiety and depression. I have overcome a lot of tough times to become the person I am today. In this book, I take you through the stages of my life. Not everything about me having autism has been difficult, but it has played a part in who I am.

Thank you for joining me on this journey through times of happiness, laughter, struggle, trauma and, most importantly, success in my career and living independently.

Blake "Crash" Priddle

---

[2]   Echolalia is the repeating (immediate or delayed) of words, sentences and/or sounds without necessarily knowing the meaning.

[3]   No disrespect to those who choose this path! It just isn't mine!

Chapter 1:

It Was the Best of Times and the Hardest of Times

**"If you've met one person with autism,
you've met one person with autism."**

Dr. Stephen Shore

My Earliest Memories

Even as a toddler, I knew I was different from other kids my age. At one Christmas dinner at my grandparents' house, out of the blue I said "delicious." This made both my parents proud that I could say such a big word but perplexed that I could not say "Good morning, Mommy." I just babbled instead of speaking.

I also went off the rails when I experienced an unexpected change. I cried inconsolably when my babysitter's son had a bubble beard—you know, bubbles from the bath that you make a beard out of. The train whistle, the coffee grinder—any loud noise freaked me out.

My parents said I was a "normal" baby, but at about eighteen months I started to detour from *typical* developmental milestones. So, let's begin with my dad's take on fatherhood and me as a baby, followed by my mom's reflections on my early years. I remember things well as a toddler aged two and up, as do many family and friends, and these are shared in this chapter.

In the Beginning

Before I came along, my parents were childless by choice. They were career-oriented, loved their free time and felt the world had enough kids. My dad (Ted) said that they were also afraid of having a physically- or intellectually-disabled child because they didn't think they had the skills and internal strength to raise one. Well, nature surprised them! In May of 1993, Jo (my mom) was pregnant, and she and my dad passed through the typical phases of prospective parents: excitement, fear, denial, selfishness, acceptance, joy.

After the initial shock subsided, they started reading the latest approaches for raising a child. Dad doesn't remember having access to any resources written on strategies for raising a disabled child, but like most parents, they wouldn't have felt the need to read these anyway.

What My Dad Remembers

I arrived! My mom had a difficult induced delivery three weeks earlier than my due date. The umbilical cord was around my neck, which my dad said caused a flurry of activity around the delivery room. I apparently struggled to breathe and had a very low Apgar score.[4] I spent the first five days in the Neonatal Critical Care Unit recuperating from pneumothorax (tear of the lung).

My dad said that it seemed like an eternity waiting to be able to go and see me. This is what he recalled:

> As you can imagine, many thoughts were going through our heads. What happened? Why did it happen? What's going to happen? Finally, after twelve LONG hours, the nurse told us that Blake was stable enough that we could see him but not touch or hold him. It was scary. Blake looked so vulnerable with tubes and wires attached to his little body. After thirty-six hours, we could finally hold him and Jo could start breastfeeding.

Going Home: My parents are voracious readers. My dad said, "You can read and research and listen to all the advice about raising a child, but it does not prepare you for the reality!" The nurses must have thought, *Poor Blake!* My mom and dad didn't know how to dress me and properly secure me in the car seat without help. And get this: they drove home slowly from the hospital because they knew that my grandparents were on their way to our house to help them. My Gramps and Grandma Roseanne stayed almost a month!

---

[4] The Apgar is a quick test done on a newborn at one and five minutes after birth to determine how well the baby tolerated the birthing process and how well he or she is doing outside the womb.

My First Year: Although I had a rough beginning, I made up for it once I got home. I'm told I ate and slept well and GREW! My baby calendar shows me "off the growth charts"—topping thirty pounds at twelve months.

"My fondest memory of Blake's first year was the bond I formed with him," my dad said. "He always wanted me to rock him to sleep and this became a very special moment for me. I often wondered if this bond was formed early as I was the first parent to be able to hold him after he was born."

Optimism, Denial or Ignorance (Or a Combination of All Three)

My dad's perspective on when I started to show autistic-like early signs differed from my mom's a bit:

> As Blake continued to grow and develop, Jo became a bit concerned that he was not meeting some milestones, particularly language development. He was also exhibiting some sensory disintegration where he'd zone out and be off in his own world; plus, loud noises and changes in routine freaked Blake out. My mom (Grandma Dot) explained to us that we all develop differently. I remember her saying, "Ted, we thought you'd never talk and then when you started, we thought you'd never shut up." Therefore, I had more of a "wait and see" attitude. Jo, however, was more concerned and started to research how we might best address these issues.

It wasn't all doom and gloom. Dad said I exhibited uncanny abilities like hearing the train coming ten minutes before everyone else, reciting highway signs I'd only seen once months before, and knowing which shoes belonged to which guests, to name a few. I had challenges and gifts just like any kid.

What My Mom Remembers

Apparently, my infancy was pretty standard fare. I went through my baby calendar that chronicles my development and found that I met my early developmental milestones—sleeping, eating, engaging, growing, cuddling—like a "normal" baby (we'll talk about the word "normal" in Chapter 5).

My mom was thrilled that I inherited her sleeping gene. By nine weeks of age, I was sleeping through the night and never missed a two-hour nap. So, unlike many on the spectrum, sleeping has never been a problem. As I got older, I tended to get up early, but sleeping at night was never an issue. Also, my gastrointestinal system never gave me grief as a baby, kid or adult, so I never had to endure any dietary tricks.

At seven months, I crawled, drank from a cup and used my fingers to eat. By eight months I was climbing stairs, playing fetch with our two labs, Nik and Kali, and waving bye. At nine months, I responded to my name, pointed to body parts (even poking Jami—my sister from another mother—in the eye to show her "eye"), and I said a few words: "outside," "snow" and "Sara."

At eleven months, I responded to "no," played peekaboo, loved books and turned pages on my own. One fairly odd thing I did was walk on my tiptoes. My mom wondered if this was an early clue even though "normal" kids did that. At twelve months, unlike my mom, I loved to push the vacuum while it was on loudly. This didn't last long as I soon developed a fear of the vacuum.

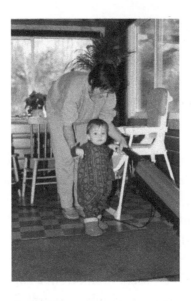

Loved vacuuming when I was one year old

I asked my mom, "When did you first think I had autism?" She told me she has been asked that question a million times and answering it never gets old. A whole lot of therapists, physicians and well-meaning friends and acquaintances have and continue to ask this question to her, and she always took it as an opportunity to engage and educate. She said that her short answer is, "When you were about two years old," but here is the long answer!

Is This "Normal" or Typical Development?

Around age two, Blake seemed to show idiosyncratic behaviour: ear covering and panic with loud noises; repetitive play that if interrupted, caused grief. Stuff that, at the time, seemed like typical toddler "terrible twos," however, as patterns emerged, we started to wonder.

Apparently, many of my developmental signs were typical, others not so much. I presented with four "early signs."

Early Sign Number 1: Unexpected Loud Noises

Everyone has a fear of something, and every child has their own fears. Some kids are afraid of the dark, while others are afraid of monsters under the bed or in the closet. I was never really bothered by the thought of monsters living under my bed, but the things that scared me the most were loud noises and certain social situations.

As a child, sudden and unexpected loud noises were especially frightening for me; even noises that other people didn't consider loud scared me. I was afraid to visit the home of our family friend Jane. We were good friends, so I wasn't afraid of her or her family, but I was afraid of the grandfather clock in the dining room. I remember eating supper at their place one time and when the clock chimed, I stopped cold because I was in shock. I wondered why the noise didn't bother everyone else, but because my hearing was so sensitive it sounded like Big Ben was ringing right next to my ears! After that experience I was afraid to go back to Jane's place. The only way I would go into the house was if someone assured me the clock was off. As I got a little older, I was ashamed that I was afraid of a clock, but it felt good to know that people around me understood my fears and didn't think I was weird.

Other loud noises that bothered me were things like the vacuum cleaner, the lawnmower, public toilets and the horn from the paper mill that was close to our house. Whenever my parents used the coffee grinder without preparing me, I would cover my ears and start crying out of fear. Mom and Dad soon learned to prepare me! The sound of the lawnmower was just too loud for me to handle, so my parents could not cut the grass, something I think my dad was thankful for. (By the way, our grass did get cut, but we would hire someone to cut the grass when we were out of town.)

Whenever I used a public washroom, someone else had to flush the toilet because they were often a lot louder than the toilets at home. I also hated the sounds of the hand dryers, so instead of using them, I would dry my hands on my shirt or pants. Often, I would use the bathroom at home before going out and hope I didn't have to go to a public washroom. It was the same thing with the bathrooms at school. I would try to avoid using them.

Thunderstorms were also difficult to deal with. Much like other loud noises, thunder sounded a lot louder to me than it did to most children. I needed my parents to help me go to sleep during a storm. They used to tell me thunder was just angels bowling. Now, I find the sound of thunder to be relaxing if it isn't too loud. If it is, I sing the "Thunder Song" from the movie *Ted*.

I managed to overcome my fear of loud noises because I was exposed to them gradually and developed a tolerance. People's understanding of my discomfort also helped. If you have a child who has a fear of loud noises, one of the best things to do is prepare them as much as you can for situations such as a party or a concert or when you are going to use loud equipment. Using earplugs or earmuffs is okay, but some people believe it's not a good idea to use them all the time because this could mess up the sensory inputs in the ears, and the child may not develop a tolerance for loud noises. If I had worn hearing protection all the time, I may still be afraid of loud noises today. Take time to find out what noises bother your child and help them to slowly overcome their fears with gradual exposure. It is best not to surprise them with loud noises.

Early Sign Number 2: Difficulty with Change in Routine

Changes were very difficult to handle as a toddler. Unexpected changes really hurt me inside. There are many examples of this, some of which I remember and will share, and others I will let my friends and family share.

The Barney Incident

In order to expose me to more kids my age and learn to socialize, my mom took the recommendation of a speech-language pathologist and drove me to a day care seventy kilometres from home one day a week. As a toddler, I have to say, day care was not one of my favourite places.

One day we all gathered around the TV to watch a movie because it was a raining. The movie was *Barney Live! In New York City*, a kid's movie that most nineties' kids loved but probably made their parents cringe. It was one of my favourite movies, and I always watched the whole seventy-five minutes without taking a break. Everyone in my life knew not to turn the TV off unexpectedly while it was on. However, the day-care workers turned it off just a few minutes before the end right when "Twinkle Twinkle Little Star" was on (yes, even now I remember when they turned the TV off!). I waited for a second to see if they would turn it back on, but they didn't. They had us all leave the room, which was traumatic for me. Within seconds, I started crying and screaming uncontrollably. This lasted for over two hours. The workers didn't know what was wrong, and I didn't have the words to tell them. Whenever I had these kinds of meltdowns it felt like a panic attack, something I could not escape from. Eventually, they called my mom because they thought I was sick.

When my mom arrived, she asked when I had started crying, and one of the workers said that we had been watching a movie. Mom asked if we had watched the whole movie, to which they said "no." That is when she understood. She knew that because I normally watched movies to the end, I would have a major meltdown if it was cut short— not a *typical* toddler temper tantrum. The people at the day care soon understood, and the caregivers learned to prepare me for these kinds of changes. As I got older, I no longer needed to be as prepared ahead of time, but having people understand that my needs were different made my life as a child more comfortable.

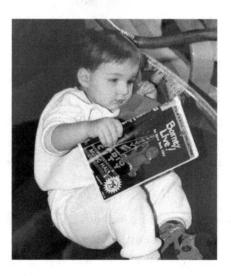

**One of my favourite videos as a toddler
caused a meltdown at day care!**

My play was predominantly *Thomas the Tank Engine* with little imaginative changes, and mostly lining up of trains. I loved to re-enact and repeat entire shows although no one could understand a word of my "jargon." It's common knowledge that many people with autism are fans of *Thomas the Tank Engine*. When it came to playing with my toy trains, I felt like I was in a safe place. From what I remember, I did allow some people to play with me, but I remember one friend telling me I didn't like it when the trains were removed from the special line I put them in. Lanny, our family friend, recalled, "One of my first memories of Blake is him playing with his trains. Before I knew anything about autism, I tried to play with him and moved his trains around. Blake was not very happy with me! He was polite, as always, but obviously very agitated."

The New Car

When I was a toddler, long before my autism diagnosis, my parents decided we needed a new car. They had driven a Ford Explorer since I was a baby, and there was something about it that I loved. One day we went for a drive and my dad pointed to our new Subaru Legacy.

"Here's our new car!" he said excitedly.

Most kids would not have been affected by this, but I was. I was silent for a few minutes, mainly because I was in shock. When it sank in that I was never going to ride in the Explorer again I broke down and cried inconsolably. My parents hadn't told me we were getting a new car ahead of time, and being surprised like that was really difficult. It soon became clear to my folks that I could not handle unexpected changes the way typical kids can.

Jami, one of my babysitter's daughters, remembered the new car story as well:

> I remember one morning Ted was dropping Blake off at our house first thing and Blake was crying really hard. His little face was red and he was trying to catch his breath. You know when you are SO upset that you can't really talk properly? Sara and I were sitting on the steps waiting for him. We were concerned and wondered

why Blake was crying. Ted explained that Blake was upset because they had gotten a new car. Blake didn't want a new car, didn't like that his routine had changed, and now his parents were driving in a different car. At the time we thought it was cute, but now looking back, we see that it was a real struggle for Blake.

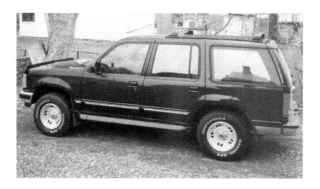

Hard to say goodbye to my first car!

Routine with the Adams Family

While my parents were at work, I spent a lot of my time with Vicki Adams, my caregiver, her husband Bim, and their kids Kelly, Jami, Sara and Cam. The entire Adams family worked hard to ensure we had a solid routine before and after school, but at times I would be thrown off. Sara remembered:

> Blake tried so hard to cope when the routine changed unexpectedly, something that often happened in a house of four school-aged kids. He would pace and repeat, "It's okay, going to sit on step." The pacing seemed like a pull for him to grasp the next step to an unfamiliar routine. Repeating, pacing and head down without focus would take over. Vicki would calmly repeat, "Blake, it's okay. Stop and sit," and she would describe what was going to happen next. She'd say, "No bus," or, "Off to the mall for toast."

I would pace when I became anxious and pace or skip if I got excited. My caregivers understood that this was my way of dealing with my emotions whether it was nervousness or happiness. Now I know it's one of my stims.[5]

Another example of my difficulty with changes comes from Vicki, who told my mom about an incident that occurred as we were walking into the mall:

> Out of nowhere, Blake started to freak out and flatten to the floor. I would not put up with that kind of tantrum, so back into the van we went. I realized later that I had turned in the opposite direction to run an errand before going for our daily breakfast at the mall food counter. The meltdown was Blake expressing how the inexplicable change in routine did not make sense in his world.

Jami, who was like a sister to me, recalled, "Everything was routine with Blake. If his routine was off so was his behaviour. Now that I am a parent, I know this is true for most kids. The difference I realize now, is that sometimes I remember Blake getting really, really upset and almost inconsolable."

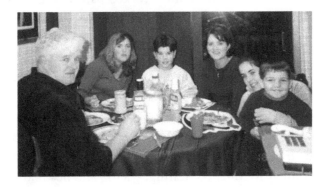

My second family: the Adams family *(courtesy V. & B. Adams)*

---

[5]   A self-stimulatory behaviour marked by a repetitive action or movement of the body (such as repeatedly hand flapping, pacing) and a protective response to less predictable environmental stimuli that some can be overly sensitive to.

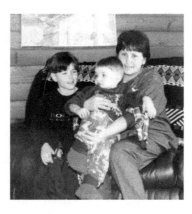

My babysitter (saviour!) Vicki and brother
from another mother, Cam

My mom told me that when they looked back on the myriad meltdowns, they began to recognize patterns emerging, "What we were witnessing, although we didn't piece it together at the time, was Blake's need for routine and sameness," she said.

Early Sign Number 3: Idiosyncratic Language

As a baby, I had lots of ear infections so I took a lot of antibiotics. My parents thought this might be why I was showing speech delays, but my hearing tests showed normal hearing. Dad said, "This did not ease our angst about Blake's language delay and sensory challenges." Apparently, I spoke in my own jabbering language. When I played with my toys, I would verbalize with what they later labelled as "jargon." He remarked, "We later came to believe, that in Blake's own language, he was actually reciting episodes of his favourite TV shows, *Thomas the Tank Engine* and *Theodore Tugboat.*"

I have always been a big fan of movies and TV shows. They played a big part in how I learned to communicate. I liked *Thomas the Tank Engine* and *Theodore Tugboat* because boats and trains are predictable, and both shows were shot on sets that didn't have any background distractions. For example, the trains started and ended at the station and there wasn't a lot of moving detail in the background. The focus was on the trains' faces, which were the only things that moved.

When it came to communication, I really enjoyed repeating lines from both shows with my Thomas and Theodore toys. I would repeat the lines, narrate the story the same way the narrators did, only in my own jargon, and sometimes I would have the entire story memorized. Now I tell stories for a living, and who knows, maybe one day I could become a narrator for a kids' show.

I took comfort in repeating lines from Disney films and TV commercials even if I didn't know what they meant. As I got older, friends told me they found this trait fascinating because it was something they could never do. Repeating lines from TV shows and movies helped to develop my speech in the long run.

I struggled with communicating the same way other people learn to speak. I often could not find the right words to tell people what I wanted or needed. Repeating words and phrases that I heard was something I did throughout my childhood. One time we were going to a Swiss Chalet restaurant but it was too busy to get a table, so Bim said, "Swiss Chalet will be nuts." I ended up using this phrase for years whenever I didn't want to go to a specific restaurant my parents picked out. Today I still occasionally repeat phrases like this.

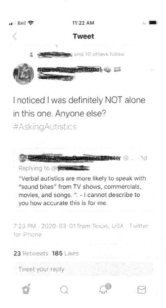

A tweet that echoes how I learned to communicate

Vicky and Bim recalled their early days learning to understand how to communicate with me. "Blake was a happy eight-month-old with an infectious belly laugh when he came into our family. When he started to speak as a toddler he jabbered constantly. Vicki would say if you recorded Blake and then slowed down the tape, 'I bet he is actually saying words.' He would carry on quite the conversation."

My "sister" Sara also recalled these times fondly:

> We all loved playing with Blake, getting him to smile and playing with him in the Jolly Jumper. I can remember Blake jumping and smiling and laughing in that thing. My mom was his primary caregiver, but my dad loved having Blake around too. Lots of times Blake would sit on his knee and they would eat their lunch together. When someone from Dad's work called in on Dad's radio, Blake would say, "Star command, come in!" (from *Toy Story*).

These early language idiosyncrasies were concerning to my parents:

> We noticed that the way Blake "communicated"— some might say "when he didn't communicate"—was the BIG EARLY SIGN. He never lost his first words, which often occurs with autism. Rather, his speech and language were simply indecipherable compared to similar-aged kids.
>
> Also: hand flapping, tippytoe walking, tactile sensory aversion to tags, collars, zippers, jeans, wool, long sleeves and loud unexpected noises, different smells or brands of pizza sauce. We felt that if Blake couldn't communicate with the outer world, it would be catastrophic.

So that's what they focused on. My mom read everything she could get her hands on (before the internet was available) and hired private speech-language pathologists (SLPs). They needed to unpack the complex and mystical way we typically learn language skills to begin to apply this for my sake:

> Before Blake was born, I never gave any thought to how each of us learns language. We just intuitively begin to reach and exhibit developmental milestones from "Dadda, Momma, bird, want juice, I want juice…."

> The title of this book, *Good Morning, Blake,* reflects the huge undertaking we all had before us to see Blake become an engaged social person.

Echolalia

My parents took me to a weekly toddler/parent Saturday morning YMCA play session—a gym full of chaos. At circle time, parents sat behind their squirming kid. Each toddler was prompted to say their name out loud. When it came to my turn, I echoed "Darryl" because that was the kid's name who sat next to me.

Echo. Echo. Echo.

So, in her usual manner, my mom found some literature to understand this unusual way of communicating. She said the need "to build on this so that Blake could communicate and not just parrot" became her new obsession.

Pronoun Reversals

> Once Blake began to use two words together (which took months of work), we had to teach him to use "I" rather than "you." So, when Blake wanted juice, he had to learn to say, "I want juice" not "You want juice." He worked very hard for over a year to get his pronouns right.

One of my earliest memories was when I was given a tough choice by my dad. Often, he would not describe the choice for me in detail. Whatever it was, he would just say, "Choose one or the other." It was torture for me as it was like playing a game where if I got the wrong answer, I would lose all my money. I would literally say, "One" hoping I had made the right choice. Then I would worry that I made the wrong choice, so I would say, "No, no, the other!" If Dad had given me the choices in better detail rather than simple speech, making a choice would have been easier for me.

I had trouble understanding words that little kids understand. Even as an adult there are still lots of "kids' words" I fail to comprehend. I remember telling a schoolyard supervisor about someone breaking a minor rule, and she told me I was being a "tattletale." I had no idea what these two words meant. I assumed that it meant I was lying, so I told her I was telling the truth. She looked at me instead and said, "Okay, maybe you don't understand what being a 'tattletale' means." She tried to explain, but she didn't do a good job because I still didn't understand.

In contrast, there were many words I understood that most kids did not. One time, the teacher was lecturing us or saying something I really did not want to hear, and I said out loud, "I am starting to get irritated." The word "irritated" is normally one only adults use, not children. My brain was wired differently than most kids.

Unlocking the Mysteries of Language

Finding the words to communicate was a struggle even as my vocabulary increased. I would hear words and speech patterns that ordinary people used every day, but I did not understand them. My mom knows a lot about speech and language because my delay forced her to learn. She has a lot of opinions and knowledge on the subject. Here she is talking about unlocking the mysteries of language:

> Kids on the spectrum are often known for their pedantic voice. I had to look up that word the first time a SLP said it. It means speaking like a little professor or sounding overly formal. Blake's intonation varied between being singsong-like and flat during the first six to eight years of his life. Singsong, because in our efforts to get him to talk we asked questions all the time and

over-emphasized words. For example, I'd say to Ted at the dinner table:

"Does Daddy want some more pizza?"

It sounded overly contrived, like I was on a sitcom and "more pizza?" would be in a raised intonation and louder.

Ted would respond, "Yes, I'd like more pizza please."

So, Ted would loudly over-emphasize "Yes, I'd" in the hope that, through modelling, when I next asked Blake the same question, he would respond, "Yes, I'd like...."

By the way, this took hundreds of tries.

Dinnertime was speech therapy in action—exhausting beyond reason. Actually, what is particularly striking when I think back, is that almost every interaction we had with Blake from age two to eighteen required me to have an internal dialogue of how and what exactly I'd say before I said it out loud. In retrospect, it might be similar to how one chooses words more carefully when speaking with someone who is an English as a Learned Language (ELL) student or uses augmentative and alternative communication methods.

It was extra work that typical kids don't generate for their parents, and unless you have a kid with a severe communication disorder you will never understand just how difficult this was.

I had difficulty grasping prepositions when I was a little kid. Words like "under," "over," "behind" and the more abstract "if" took years to master. The word "if" is simple in its spelling but is fraught with misunderstanding. How do you teach the meaning of "if"? Here's my mom with an example of how they tried:

> Blake loved going to camp and swimming at Tobacco Lake on Manitoulin Island. As the weekend approached, we'd say, "If it rains, we won't go to camp and swim." Blake just comprehended "we aren't going." No comprehension of "if." "If" requires a higher order of abstract and inferential reasoning. It took Blake years to learn this. Misunderstanding "if" statements almost always resulted in meltdowns that could last for hours.

My parents told me they spent thousands of dollars on speech therapy for me to learn the "Five Ws"—what, where, when, who, why. They said they'd get mad whenever they heard other parents complaining that their kid was always asking them "Why, why, why?" I endured years of language therapy sessions to master what most intuitively learn on their own. It clearly paid off as I have asked the Five Ws many times in my career as a journalist. What an accomplishment!

Scaffold

When I was about six years old, a developmental pediatrician told my parents that they would be my "scaffold." I didn't know what a scaffold was, so I ignored the conversation. Here's my mom's recollection of that appointment:

> In time, this word "scaffold" would ring true. So did the analogy of speaking a foreign language—you know, when you are in a foreign country and the home language is one you don't know. You automatically pull out the translation book or app, and fumble for the words, pronunciation, tone, pace of speech. I know a wee bit of French and Spanish, but when my French-speaking friends talk, I immediately miss half the conversation and eventually tune out or ask them to slow down and spell it out. So when Blake was young

that's what I learned we had to do. When talking to Blake, we had to pause, pick words carefully and slowly and then state a question or comment.

During an interaction with others (Grandma, teacher, peer), I would be at the ready to scaffold when I could see the attempted conversation going sideways.

"Blake, Grandma means, 'Do you want soup now?' not, 'Do you like soup?'"

Simple misreads of basic interactions, multiplied by the thousands.

Difficulty with transition of any sort, coupled with significant semantic and pragmatic language deficits, made us realize that Blake was marching to the beat of a different drum compared to his peers.

Early Sign Number 4: Hyper- and Hypo-Sensitivities

People on the autism spectrum have different kinds of sensory issues; no two are alike. Having a difficult time with loud noises was one of many sensory issues I had as a child. But that was just the tip of the iceberg. There were some things that didn't bother me sensorially that other autistic people can't stand, and there were things I didn't like that didn't bother others on the spectrum.

Get This off Me! And Turn on the AC!

My earliest memory is when I suddenly could not wear certain pieces of clothing that I was able to wear before. For example, I was not able to wear shirts with collars because they felt itchy. Buttons felt like I was wearing pebbles and were uncomfortable. I also could not wear pants with flies. So, for the longest time I would just not wear things that I couldn't stand the feel of, and at the same time, I would see other people wearing clothing that I didn't like and wonder why it didn't bother them. I can wear these items now, but I leave the formal attire to formal occasions! The one thing I did not like then (and still don't) are tags on the back of shirts or pants. I always have to remove them before I put them on, otherwise they drive me insane.

I also did not like the feel of certain things in my hands or on my skin. I had sensitive skin, which often meant I had to have cream put on me. I hated that more than anything. It was always a battle for my parents to put any kind of cream on me because that was far worse than being itchy or having a sunburn. My parents didn't understand why I was so bothered, but as I got older, I had the words to tell them that whenever they put cream on me it felt like they were putting honey on my skin. My mom understood right away because whenever she gets even a little bit of honey on her hand she must clean it off right away. It felt good to know I could finally tell my parents how I felt. I still dislike putting cream on, but I can handle it a lot better now than I did back then.

My sensory abilities were a little odd in some cases. I enjoyed the feeling of mud in my hands, but finger paints were a different story. I remember finger-painting for the first time in kindergarten, and I didn't like the way it felt on my hands, so I used the paper that they gave me to wipe it off. Somehow, I liked the way it felt when someone would paint my hands and feet with a paint brush because when they did that, I felt relaxed and almost fell asleep. Perhaps it was because the amount of paint on my hands was controlled. Also, we were just making prints, so I knew it wouldn't be on my hands or feet for very long, which made me feel a bit better. I also did not enjoy the feeling of pumpkin pulp or tree sap on my hands.

I had a very high tolerance for the cold from a young age and have always loved the water. I have no issue swimming in cold water (12°C Lake Superior in September!), and even though people would tell me that the water was too cold I didn't care—I enjoyed it! Some kids on the spectrum don't like getting wet, but this is a good example of how I enjoyed something that others may find uncomfortable.

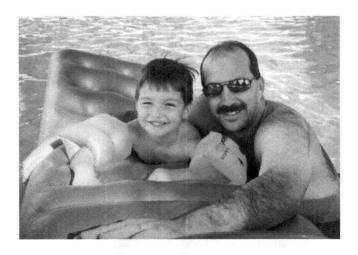

If the water is cold, I'm in it!

People who know me will tell you I hate being hot, in any season, because I get heat rashes. Many contributors to this book wrote something about me wearing no layers in the winter or swimming in frigid water. My mom got a stern letter from the principal one time because I arrived at school with no winter clothes on. Mom told me she used to drive around the schoolyard after lunch recess to find my hoodies pealed off and tossed. She told me that she regularly rummaged through the school office Lost and Found box for my mitts, hats and hoodies. Eliza, a lifelong family friend, summed up how much I love the cold: "I can remember numerous holidays on Faraway Road where all of us would be outside, bundled up in multiple layers, hats, gloves, snow pants, boots, handwarmers, trying to get warm by the fire, and Blake would be wearing a T-shirt and wind pants and not bothered at all!"

I had a very high tolerance for pain from a very young age. I liked to walk along the driveway curb, but one day while I was with Bim, I stumbled and slipped to the pavement, scraping both knees badly. Bim ran to help me up and give me a hug and said, "Blake, are you all right?" Apparently, I just gritted my teeth and said, "Okay Bim." Bim was amazed at my lack of a reaction. Any of his kids would have been crying profusely, especially when they saw blood, but not me.

Lastly, I grew to have many food hypersensitivities. The smell, texture, taste and temperature would throw me into a tizzy. As a toddler

I started out as an adventurous eater, then I became super picky for many years and had a limited diet, and now I am an adventurous eater again! Pizza still remains my favourite food!

Nothing Green on a Pepperoni Pizza

Generally, people with autism are different when it comes to eating, and lots of people on the spectrum have difficulties with food. We have true sensory issues! For instance, some may only eat one kind of food while others will eat everything, even things that are not edible. When I was a baby and a toddler, I ate just about anything my parents and babysitter fed me, but I became quite picky around three years old. My mom wasn't too concerned because she felt it was normal for preschoolers to go through a picky eating phase. Over time, my picky eating became a hypersensitivity issue. Foods that I used to be able to eat were no longer edible to me. Chicken pot pie and lasagna, two foods I often begged my babysitter to make me, made me want to vomit if I even looked at them. The only way I would eat meat is if it was taken off the bones. The food the day-care centre served was out of the question, mainly because it wasn't the same food I was familiar with. I wouldn't try foods that most kids love, like dinosaur chicken nuggets, because they were new to me.

I also struggled with eating certain foods they served in my kindergarten class. If I saw we were being served something I didn't like, I would often start crying because I didn't have the words to tell them that I didn't like the food. I was afraid I would be forced to eat something I didn't like, people would get mad at me for not eating it or I would be punished. The teachers and the lunch supervisors soon realized this, and they didn't force me to eat things I didn't like, which made me feel better about eating at school.

As I got older, I developed additional food aversions. I could no longer eat old cheddar cheese, Kraft Dinner or brown bread. If food wasn't exactly the same as I was used to in terms of smell, taste, texture and temperature, I couldn't eat it. Being forced to try new foods was scary for me and would often result in a meltdown or a minor panic attack. I would rather go hungry than eat foods I hated. Now I eat pretty much anything except for baked beans, any kind of pasta, and gelatin because of texture sensitivities.

This story always comes to mind when I share stories about my picky eating experiences as a child. I was five years old in the summer of 1999. My parents and I drove out of town for a family friend's wedding. The moment the wedding started I knew it was going to be a long day. I was bothered because I had to wear a dress shirt with a collar, something my parents knew I hated but made me wear anyway. I still could not understand why the buttons on shirts didn't bother other people. It felt like having needles stuck into me. In addition, it was super hot that day, which made me even more uncomfortable, and I had to sit in a church pew during the wedding. I felt like a ticking time bomb.

After a long wedding reception with lots of noise, I was ready to call it a night. But as luck would have it, the grown-ups had other plans. We ate supper at a fancy restaurant, one of those places that kids hate to go to because they are expected to sit up straight and be on their best behaviour. From what I recall, there was not a lot on the menu I would like except for pizza, and at the time I would only eat pepperoni and cheese pizza. We had to wait a really long time for our food, so I was ready to lose it.

The next part of the story is somewhat disputed between Mom and me. When the pizza finally arrived, it was not pepperoni pizza at all; it was a cheese pizza that was caked in parsley. The idea of having any vegetables or herbs on a pizza, especially if they were green, would not do it for me at the age of five. With everything that I'd had to endure that day, I went into a full-blown meltdown. Normally, if I didn't want to eat something that I didn't think I would like, I would just say "no," but not this time.

My mom assumed I was just acting up, and boy was she mad. While I was screaming and crying, Mom grabbed me and said to me in a loud voice that I was ruining the dinner. That certainly didn't help because I felt like I was having a panic attack, not a temper tantrum. Things really got out of hand when Mom picked me up and took me out of the restaurant and started speed walking to our room. I was scared because I thought I was going to be punished. Instead of being punished, my parents went out and got me the type of pizza I love to eat.

Sometimes I look back on this night and feel bad about what I did, but Mom and Dad said it was all part of growing up. This episode helped them understand I was tapped out with too much stimulation and change. When I asked why I was put through these situations, they would tell me that if I was never taken outside my comfort zone, I would not have overcome any challenges that used to make me uncomfortable. Once I was diagnosed with ASD, my parents and other people understood me better and were able to help me deal with similar situations in a different way.

Since we have to eat a bunch of times every day, mealtimes could have turned into a battleground because I had lots of aversions, but as people began to understand me and I became better at communicating, we figured out what worked best for all of us. Here are friends and family members' recollections around the dinner table.

Vicky Miron was a friend of my mom's, my respite worker, and the mother of my autistic friend, Jakob. She remembered:

> One of the earliest battles we had was dinner time. Blake was very apprehensive to even look at new food. Oh my gosh, how dare I suggest he eat a chicken drumstick? After a long struggle and lots of tears, I persuaded Blake to look at the food while telling him next time it will be to hold it in his hand. He had a full meltdown, pacing the hallway, wiping his eyes and telling me I was just not nice.

> The following week we had the same encounter. Blake decided he could look at the food but he wouldn't taste it. Then the following week he put it in his mouth and could spit it in the garbage. I would always make something that he did like, and I told him that the food he did not like would be on the plate as well. I think it took a month before he decided to eat the chicken on a bone and it became something he enjoyed.

Blake got used to me challenging him because it didn't take him long before he would pace and wipe his eyes and tell me while pacing that he needed time. It was cute how he resigned himself to the fact that there was going to be something about our visits that would challenge him.

Every family has its own mealtime rules and regular foods they serve. My parents refused to make mealtime a battle. They figured that since I was off the growth charts and taking vitamins, I was healthy and might eventually expand my limited choice of foods (which, as you will read in later chapters, has definitely happened). When I was transitioning from toddler to preschooler, my mom said I went eighteen months without eating a vegetable except the occasional frozen peas, but I ate tons of fruit. The only fresh vegetable I would eat at the time was steamed fiddleheads!

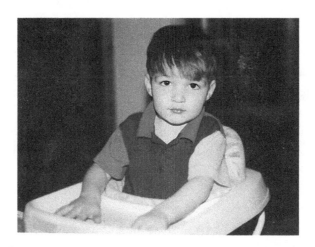

Waiting to eat something I was familiar with and liked!

Lanny, a dear family friend, recalled my parents trying to get me to sample different foods, especially vegetables, many times. "One time Blake stayed with us, I made pasta without realizing he didn't (and still doesn't) like its texture. He was older, and very polite about it, but he didn't eat much that night!"

My good friend Eliza said, "I also always found it so strange that Blake hates pasta. I realize this is completely ironic coming from someone who used to be an incredibly picky eater, but my inner carb lover could never comprehend it! Now that I am older and understand that it is a texture thing, I can relate."

I ate all the other food groups daily but without much variety. Cooked deli ham sliced into small squares (not big), extra old cheddar cheese (not medium), and yogurt in tubes (not cups), seemed to be staples alongside pizza (only two brands were tolerable). I ate other food, but when I couldn't handle the smell, texture, temperature or look, I would gag and the meal would often not end well.

My Aunt Helen and Uncle Randy always cooked amazing meals. They were stricter around my cousins' food choices, so I can imagine that when we came to visit they wondered why my parents seemed to cater to my peculiar eating habits when I was little. Here were their recollections:

> When it came to sitting down to dinner, Blake was a picky eater. Cooked veggies were not Blake's favourite. Veggies had to be served raw for Blake to eat them. We were at the cottage one summer, and Blake was spending a few days with us while Jo and Ted were working. After a day of swimming and playing in the sun, it was dinner time. We sat down to BBQ chicken, potatoes and cooked green beans. We tried endlessly to convince Blake to just try one green bean—even the kids tried—but there was no way Blake was going to eat that bean.

> When Blake liked a food, he would eat it like there was no tomorrow. Some of the foods Blake loved as a kid were grapes, pancakes and bacon. Ah, Blake who ate all the bacon!

My mom's friend Lee, who is a pediatric registered dietitian (RD), noticed a few things about my eating when I was a toddler. These were her reflections:

> The first time it hit home for me that there might be some "red flags" with Blake's development was in a meeting with other RDs when Blake's mom said she was concerned about his change in eating habits as a toddler. One of our RD colleagues, who was older and had three kids of her own, told Blake's mom she was overreacting and not to worry. But I had worked in clinical pediatrics with cases of feeding disorders and children with special needs for a few years. I was also a mom who was dealing with issues of picky eating, iron deficiency anemia, food intolerances and suspected attention deficit hyperactivity disorder (ADHD), so I was pretty sure we shouldn't disregard Blake's mom's intuition.

A few years ago, I wrote a blog for an autism website that included the following tips on dealing with picky eaters:

- Realize that it is "normal" for young kids to go through a stage of picky eating. Kids with autism have extra-strong sensory abilities. This means that the smells, tastes, textures and even the temperatures of foods are magnified much more for us than neurotypical people.
- Never force or bribe your child to eat any food.
- Try the same method my parents tried with me. Have them at least put the unfamiliar food in their mouth. If they don't like it, they have the option to spit it out.
- Slowly expose a new food. Start with serving a food that smells or tastes new on their plate.
- The next time you introduce a new food, put a small amount on their plate and tell them that they do not have to try it. The next few times the new food is served at a meal, if your child is

in a good mood, suggest that they smell it. If they like the smell, they just might try it.

- See your doctor or dietitian if you have any concerns about your child's eating habits.

These steps would have made my experience with food somewhat easier, but kids don't come with an instruction manual, even if my mom was a dietitian!

Forming the Beat of My Own Drum

Many people who have known me since birth or my early years have observed my idiosyncratic behaviour. Some shared their concerns and observations with my parents at the time, some have shared them over the years, and some have just shared them when I asked them to for this book.

Lee, the pediatric dietitian whom I quoted earlier, wrote that since I was huge for my age, people assumed I was older than I really was and expected more from me:

> This has nothing to do with ASD, but Blake was above average size (weight/length/height) as an infant/toddler and so much bigger and growing faster than my first son, who is four months older than him. That is my first recollection as a new mother. We are trained to focus on our children's growth and caloric intakes, and with Blake there was this big difference. Even as professionals, we still compare even though each child is their "own reference." And so, Blake's growth rate and size just made it more difficult for him, like most kids above the 99th percentile. It is assumed he is older and more mature, and so he should be able to behave accordingly, regardless of whether he has challenges.

And of course, the Adams family, who I spent so much time with, had lots to say about my individuality!

Sara recalled:

> Blake's early life brought a lot of joy to our family! He excelled at tasks at a young age and would repeat the action over and over, with a lot of laughter, specifically when he started to learn to walk. One time when he was in the jolly jumper, Cam dropping a tissue on his head, which he really liked the feeling of. We laughed hard, and he jumped harder and harder with excitement!
>
> At a very young age, Blake showed gentle ways and was never aggressive or mean. He struggled to pair his inflections of tone with the feeling he was exhibiting. For example, his tone would sometimes stay neutral, but he would be saying that he was sad or excited about something. His tone of voice didn't always match what he said.
>
> When something like spilling his milk happened, we could see how stuck in the action Blake became. It was hard to pull him out of it. I remember Blake repeating:
>
> "Spilt the milk, oh no. Spilt the milk, oh no."
>
> Vicki would say, "Blake, sit down and take a breath. Accidents happen," in an attempt to refocus and calm him. She was getting Blake to connect, "Yes, spills happen, but let's regroup now and move on."
>
> Blake would get stuck on a mistake, and we could see how he would struggle to recognize that it was okay, this is life and these things happen and will happen again. He needed extra assistance to help him realize these incidents were just accidents and didn't make him "bad."

The struggle was apparent for Blake. Jo was an amazing resource to help us redirect Blake to cope with these situations. Routine, repetition and familiarity were important to keep him calm and feeling safe.

This next story illustrates the beginning of my literal thinking. It is a common trait of autistic communication that can cause problems, and as people began to understand this quality in me, we all learned that I needed to be taught about the difference between abstract thinking and literal thinking. This first example must have been hard for Vicki to figure out!

Around three years old, Blake loved to go to library school every week. It was fun for Blake and he enjoyed being with all the other kids. Blake liked the movie *Toy Story* and had watched it many times with Sara and Cam. Halloween time at the library was exciting for Blake. He wanted to go as "Woody," so I got a costume for him complete with fringed vest, chaps and a leather hat. Blake looked awesome!

When it was time to go to the party, Blake was actually jumping with joy, had a big smile in his face and was jabbering a mile a minute. When we stepped out the front door Blake stopped dead in his tracks. He kept pulling me back toward the house. I didn't understand what Blake was feeling, and he kept repeating, "Vicki, car seat?" and started to cry.

I said, "Yes Blake, it's okay, honey."

I buckled him in and Blake kept anxiously saying, "Okay Vicki, okay, go, go!"

I began driving to the library wondering why Blake was so worried. It suddenly occurred to me that because Blake was dressed like Woody, he thought he was

Woody. Blake remembered from the *Toy Story* movie that Woody was dragged behind his van when he left his house. In Blake's little mind he thought I was going to tie him to the back of the van and drag him to the library!

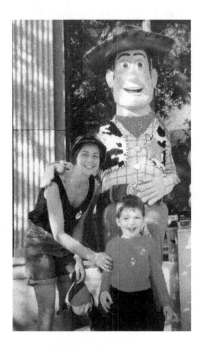

**Meeting "Woody" from *Toy Story* at
Disney World was a highlight**

Sara's brother, Cam, could write his own book about all the things we did together over the years. As he was closer in age than the Adams girls, he was like my big brother. Here's one story he remembered:

When Blake was little, he caught a muskie on a bobber. It was a small fish but special because it's not every day you catch a muskie of any size! Blake spent the whole day with the fish, taking it up and down the water slide and even bringing it through the sprinkler. We ended up naming it "Harry."

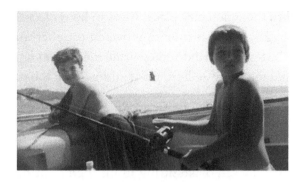

Cam and I fishing—maybe for Harry?! *(courtesy V. & B. Adams)*

From Kelly, my sister from another mother:

> I remember a social awkwardness that consisted of
> pacing and bursts of laughter…that maybe didn't fit in
> the conversation during family interactions. It didn't
> matter to me, that was Blake and he was happy…even
> making us laugh through his eyes on things that maybe
> we didn't recognize or notice! Blake would often get
> up and go to the bathroom or a quiet place. In his mind
> he needed to be by himself because he couldn't sit still
> or he would pace. As Blake got older, I noticed him
> applying his coping mechanisms and getting parental
> support if he needed time away.

All Things Trains

Many people who contributed to this book had their own train
memory of me. *Thomas the Tank Engine* played a large role when I was
little. Here's a cute story Grandma Roseanne recalled:

> Thomas the Tank was a popular toy for Blake—all
> the characters were very close to Blake. He knew all
> by name. One morning when he was three or four,
> we went to Science North in Sudbury while Jo was at
> work. Blake knew where he wanted to go, and the toy
> trains were the destination. I sat a distance away and

watched the action take place. After an hour I went over and suggested it was time to move on to other things. Well, he took my hand and escorted me back to my seat and told me "Stay"—he wasn't finished with the trains.

Shelley, a long-time family friend and speech language therapist, reflected:

> I can vividly see Blake sitting in his high chair deeply engrossed in *Thomas the Tank Engine*. There was no distracting him. Turning off the TV was not an option. Trying to converse with him was not an option. He knew every character, every scene, every action. We thought, *Wow, this kid has an incredible memory for details!* And he did. I remember noticing that when my son was with Blake, play became parallel and eye contact was almost non-existent.

> Play dates were sometimes difficult for Blake. He was over-stimulated and often needed little breaks to calm himself down. He needed to sit quietly. Talking to Blake didn't offer calm, he needed time by himself or with a Thomas video. It was sad to see how quickly he could become overwhelmed and upset. It was difficult to know how to offer him calm. But Blake never showed physical aggression; if anything, he apologized repeatedly as if somehow becoming overwhelmed was his fault. It broke my heart.

Jami, my sister from another mother, observed that when I liked something, I REALLY liked it!

> *Toy Story* and *Thomas the Tank Engine* come to mind as two things Blake loved. Again, this can also be true for any kids, as I am learning my son just loves fancy cars. The difference was that there was very little

compromise. Blake had to have everything exactly like the show, and if it wasn't then he would get upset.

I remember one time I thought I would be nice and sit down with Blake to play with his trains. I picked up the blue one and said, "Okay, I'll be Percy."

Blake very quickly corrected me and said, "No, this is Thomas."

I started playing and accidentally called it Percy again, and this upset Blake because the train's name was not Percy, it was Thomas.

In his little mind Blake was probably thinking, *Geez Jami, get it right!*

Louise Picard, a family friend, former boss and colleague of my mom's, remembered my mom telling her about a visit to a place with a real steam engine train. "Blake made quite an impression. He was on the train chattering away, and the conductor was so impressed with how knowledgeable he was. Little did he know Blake was reciting one of the *Thomas the Tank Engine* books."

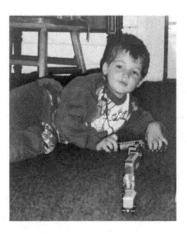

Playing with my *Thomas* trains—likely re-enacting an entire episode

Words and Actions Matter

If I was at home with no play dates, I could play for hours by myself immersed in my trains and videos. My parents say I was easy to entertain because I spent most of my time in my own world, but if you tried to get me to join another activity, I was not a happy camper. As an only child with no siblings I didn't have to share my toys and space at home. On the advice of the SLPs, in order for me to work on my social communication skills, my mom arranged play dates at our place. Here's my mom retelling a play-date scenario from when I was about four years old:

> "He's weird," remarked Blake's play date.
>
> Blake was spinning the bar stool seat around and around, oblivious to his friend in the room. *Wheel of Fortune* was in play.
>
> *Oh, well. Not how I was expecting the play date to go*, I thought. *Deep breath, Jo*. It was a teachable moment.
>
> "What do you mean by 'He's weird'?" I asked Blake's play date.
>
> "Well, Blake's playing with the stool, and I keep asking him what he's doing and he's ignoring me."
>
> "Okay. Blake is playing out a *Wheel of Fortune* scene using the stool seat as the spinner. He likes to re-enact TV and video episodes because it gives him joy and comfort," I said.
>
> I didn't know if the last bit was true, but he'd go into meltdown if we stopped him. His playmate easily absorbed this explanation and even started spinning her own stool seat! The word "weird" has always bothered me. Maybe it shouldn't, but it does.

"We prefer to say he's different," I said, "and not use the word 'weird.'"

"Why?" she asked.

"It makes it seem that you think less of Blake," I responded.

"Oh, okay!" she said.

Diagnostic Odyssey

"We all must look at life believing in all abilities and celebrating the beauty of uniqueness of all people."

Sue Nielsen, journalist

It is impossible for me to describe the long process and amount of time my parents went through trying to help me reach my potential. Before I asked my mom to write about when I received my diagnosis, I thought it was a simple doctor's appointment and *presto!* I was told I have autism. It wasn't quite as easy apparently. About all I recall is seeing lots of doctors across Ontario over the years. Nothing really stood out for me at these appointments. Most of the psychiatrists, developmental pediatricians and psychologists talked at length with my parents and generally ignored me. It's funny to think that in one pediatrician's office I was asked to catch and throw a ball. What has that got to do with autism?![6] In kindergarten, the school psychologist made me do a bunch of paper tests and peppered me with questions I had trouble answering. Here's what my mom had to say about my diagnostic odyssey:

---

[6]   Autistic folks often have gross-motor problems, such as a clumsy, uncoordinated gait; trouble with actions requiring hand-eye co-ordination (catching a ball!); and difficulties with fine motor control (no wonder I never learned how to cursive write).

Remember, this is the late nineties. There was no Dr. Google. Family doctors and many pediatricians held the belief that all kids ripen at different stages, especially boys. Valid and reliable assessment tools were not available. Early on, some well-meaning but superficially skilled folks would say, "But he shows empathy so he can't be autistic." That comment usually came after I would retell the time at toddler play group when Blake walked over to see a crying baby. So, was he showing care or simply looking for the source of the annoying noise and wanting it to stop?!

Of course, I hung on to these threads of typical behaviour, all the while knowing they were a façade and false hope. It took us many years and many labels to land on what Blake was living with.

Label or No Label, That is the Question

My parents tell me I've received a lot of labels from many professionals over the years. The following labels accumulated starting at age two:
- Semantic and pragmatic language disorder
- Non-Verbal learning disability
- Sensory disintegration disorder
- Atypical autism
- Tourette syndrome (ruled out)
- Pervasive developmental disorder – not otherwise specified (PDD-NOS)
- Asperger's syndrome
- Autism spectrum disorder
- Obsessive-compulsive disorder
- Generalized anxiety disorder
- Clinical depression

Mom and Dad agreed that labels are gateways to services and offer some understanding for those who came in contact with me. They were concerned that broadcasting me as autistic would also conjure up and reinforce ignorance, exclusion and ableism. Here's what Mom had to say about my many labels:

> Blake received other labels that came about from myriad school psychological and learning assessments. With my educational background I was able to discern how much stock to put into these assessment results and labels. Most assessments were so biased (toward neurotypical students) that the results weren't applicable to autistic students who often have executive functioning deficits. We just focused on the written comments, tips and strategies listed by the assessor.

To label or not. That is the question best answered by you and only you.

Jami said it best:

> Get educated. Understand what autism is and how it is a spectrum. It is different yet sometimes similar for every person on that spectrum. Reach out for the resources you are entitled to and advocate for the person and family with autism. Develop and surround the person and their family with a support system. There will be good days and bad days.

> These are people with autism...notice I said *people* first. Autism is a part of who they are but not the entire person. People with autism are brothers, sons, friends, teachers, radio announcers, dads, husbands, Olympians, chefs, mechanics, doctors...they are anything they want to be and so much more than a diagnosis. Don't look at the label, look at the person...but understand the label.

Good Grief or No Grief?

I was diagnosed in kindergarten, but my parents didn't tell me I had autism until I was nine years old. I asked Mom why a younger autistic family friend seemed to be non-verbal, and she told me it was because he had autism and that I have a mild case of it too. I didn't know what the new word meant, and I was a bit puzzled because I could talk and understand people for the most part, but my friend seemed to struggle more than me.

I wasn't embarrassed or ashamed; in fact, knowing helped to answer a lot of questions—like why I was going to speech camp, why it was more difficult for me to make friends, why change and making eye contact was challenging, why I had to learn idioms in therapy sessions, why my teachers used a communication book, and so on. Now I knew why, but there were still things I wasn't sure of that I would learn as time went on. I was concerned that I might not be like everyone else I went to school with—that I would be forced to be in a segregated class and wouldn't make any friends. I was determined to prove I wasn't going to let my autism negatively control my life. I decided I would always try to improve my social communication skills and not quit even if it got tough.

Grief is a topic I can't get my head around. Maybe if I was a parent…. Anyway, my mom felt it was important to share her experience of grappling with the realization that I showed differences. Unlike my dad, she went through an emotional roller coaster when I was a preschooler. Ever the academic, here's what she wrote about in learning about feelings related to a developmental disability diagnosis:

> Recent Canadian research by Stephen Gentles, David Nicholas and colleagues provided insight into the complex nature of parents accepting an autistic diagnosis.
>
> Grieving is transient and not every parent goes through it. The researchers infer that when parents get to the stage where they "know something is wrong," they begin the emotional process of releasing (and recasting)

culturally-based hopes and expectations for their child's future. They start imagining the possible long-term implications of a serious developmental disability— commonly involving milestones like university, marriage, employment and living independently.

My mom told me she has gone through this thinking process. My dad, on the other hand, has not gone through it. He tells me that he has never grieved, never had to. My mom said it's important to "acknowledge that every person, including autistic folks themselves, may or may not go through thoughts and processes that invoke grieving emotions. We must be respectful of each person's personal journey."

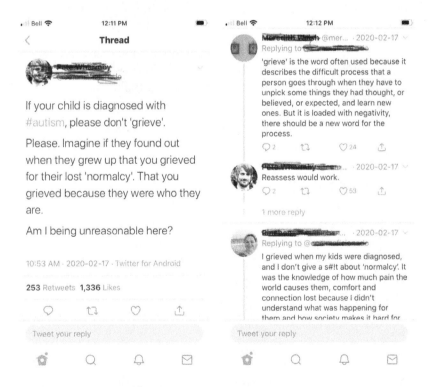

**Tweet chat illustrating the debate of
grieving for an autism diagnosis**

A few people who contributed to this book told me their feelings after I received my diagnosis.

Shelley wrote:

> As a speech therapist, I had resources on the topic of autism. I wanted to help Blake's parents, my best friends, connect the dots and try and figure out why their beautiful boy was behaving differently. I remember coming to the realization that maybe Blake was autistic. I cried. I knew that Jo and Ted suspected something. It was so difficult because we knew that the path ahead was going to be physically and mentally exhausting.

Another lifelong friend of my mom's, Laura, who was a special education elementary teacher, described meeting me for the first time when I was five months old:

> Having had three babies of my own, I must admit that I had a niggly sense that something about Blake was a bit atypical. Just an intuition, really. When holding Blake, he seemed rigid, not as cuddly as some babies, and his social interactions seemed different.

> Fast forward a few years…. I remember being so blown away by Blake's ability to recount the *Toy Story* dialogue when he was a toddler. He knew all the words, for all the characters, with proper intonation and expression. Absolutely incredible! It was also around this time that we met Blake's family at Science North. He knew all the letters on their sign. My four-year-old son, who was two years older, knew none. I remember thinking, *Blake's a genius, what's up with my kid?!*

When Jami found out I was diagnosed with autism, she had mixed feelings:

> I was ignorant and didn't really understand what autism was. I only knew the stereotypes. Jo shared some information to educate us about the autism spectrum.

I began to understand that a diagnosis is different for everyone and that many live a fulfilling life; not everyone is like the man from the movie *Rain Man.*

I was somewhat happy to hear that Blake was diagnosed with autism because at that point we could begin to understand what his brain was thinking and try our best to work with him to give him the tools he needed for support.

Kelly, my sister from another mother, remarked, "When I found out Blake had autism it did not change my love for him, it made me understand him! Acceptance is key to dealing with anyone with autism because you can learn so much about their perspective and appreciate things that you may not have noticed."

Gary, family friend recalled:

When I learned about Blake's autism it did not make me feel differently toward him in any negative way. If anything, it made me want to pay special attention, observe his interactions and pay close attention to what he had to say to make sure I could learn about what autism meant for him. How did it affect his relationships? How did he express himself? What was important to him?

My Aunt Sue reflected on her own journey upon hearing of my autism diagnosis:

I was really worried for Blake when I first learned that he was autistic, but it was because I did not have any knowledge of what that meant. I worried that he would struggle. I learned from Blake that autism is not negative, in fact it is another word for awesome—totally and utterly awesome. He is bright, funny, caring, kind and loving, and he is determined to follow his dreams. I admire and love Blake, and I am so very proud of him.

As is often the case when people learn about an autism diagnosis, most don't fully understand it. This was the case with Uncle Randy, Aunt Helen and my cousins Steven, Nick and Danielle:

> When Blake was diagnosed, we really didn't understand what autism was about. It was a learning experience for all of us. Our kids were always very inclusive with Blake, taking him to visit their friends. Gradually we learned to understand the characteristic traits he had: We understood why he paced; that he needed to know departure plans; that he would recite stories when he was in his own world; that he could recall past events right to the month, year and actual date; that he loved to impersonate people like his Uncle Randy—"Steven, Nicholas, time for bed!"

And finally, my lifelong friend Eliza recalled:

> I don't remember ever "finding out" Blake was autistic. I've known him since birth, and his family is very open about talking about autism; I just grew up knowing it. I think this is great because it made Blake's autism less of a diagnosis or a "thing" and more of just a part of who he is. It's kind of like: Blake is tall, Blake loves movies, Blake has autism. It's just something that makes him who he is.

If only more people could think like this.

Now you have a sense of what my early years were like, who I am and who my family and friends are. You will no doubt have recognized some traits in yourself or others with autism. I hope the stories have been helpful. Perhaps you are curious to learn how we all managed as I got older. I will use the next chapter to describe my elementary school years, complete with challenges and accomplishments.

Chapter 2:

From Finger Paints to Prom Dates: My Elementary School Years

"There is no such thing as common sense. If there was everyone would know everything and no one would have to learn new things."

Me

☆

Teachers Extraordinaire

I had the good fortune to have amazing teachers all through my elementary and secondary years. My parents will say that there was only one "dud" in fourteen years. This person wasn't overly harmful, just kind of ambivalent to students like me who could have benefitted from different learning strategies. This teacher thought there was only one way to teach, and if you didn't get their way, too bad.

Back in the 1990s and early 2000s, autistic kids were just beginning to be "mainstreamed" (integrated into general classrooms), usually with some special education support which happened either in a separate classroom or by withdrawal. Many of the teachers I had in primary grades did not have any training or experience with autism but were very keen to learn. They also welcomed my mom's input and together formed a great team every year fighting for what I needed and doing their best to figure it out.

In kindergarten, my first special education teacher, Deb Merchant, recalled:

> I think Blake was the first student I worked with who had an autism designation. While my knowledge was limited, Blake didn't fit my image of an autistic student. I was confident in my ability to teach students to read and do math, but I wasn't sure where to start with Blake.
>
> Getting him to engage with his peers was a major issue. He was more comfortable around adults and tended to gravitate to them, so when Blake came into the classroom

he'd greet me and require a lot of encouragement to talk to one of his peers. I remember Blake standing on the edge looking on and struggling to take the next step forward and engage with others.

He was not very athletic, so when we tried to engage him in some of the schoolyard games, he was not good at them. As a result, he wasn't keen to continue and, of course, the others weren't keen to have him on their team. I'm not sure whether that had anything to do with his athleticism or if he just hadn't spent enough time working on the skill. Did it relate to the autism or was he just not athletic like many of us?

Blake generally had a positive attitude. Despite the frustrations and anxieties, he was not an angry child. Every now and again he tried his hand at humour. Sometimes it worked, sometimes not so much—like any five- or six-year-old.

Another special education teacher of mine, Jacquie Tarnowski, reflected on a few strategies she used to help me cope:

Social journals were an ever-present part of Blake's day and seemed to give him a reference point to help him deal with situations. There were suggestions written there to help him respond to different events. We wrote many of these together.

I also remember putting a stoplight on his desk. The idea was that if he was getting worked up or was confused about an assignment, he would stop, take a moment and then ask the teacher or another student to clarify.

I remember Blake often being alone on the playground at recess in the primary grades.

I must say that when I think of Blake, I smile.

My Grade 1 teacher, Cathy Clackett, was really soft-spoken, gentle and nice. Despite having taught for many years, she told me:

> I hate to admit this, but years ago (2000-2001), I really didn't have the knowledge about autism that I should have. It was a shame that so many professional development days were spent on curriculum rather than on issues affecting our precious students!

> I noticed a few things that were different about Blake: on his first day I knew it was very stressful for him and he was having trouble coping. Blake was very quiet and he moved very slowly. The typical bounce of a Grade 1 student on day one was not there. He was terrified: new class, new teacher, new peers, new everything. Yikes! The coatroom would have been a nightmare for Blake with all the chatter and scrambling. His countenance and body language indicated fear and hesitation. He was a serious little guy! His mom was there to ease the situation and offer encouragement. She was Blake's pillar of strength (and mine as well).

> Blake internalized thoughts and fears. They would resurface and distract him or cause him to lose focus to the point where he would not know where to start or what to do next. This would cause more stress, and he would become disengaged and appear to be somewhere else. A soft touch and encouragement brought our Blake back very quickly though!

> He was a very sensitive boy. If another student was upset and hurting, so was Blake. His peers in the class, as young as they were, recognized that compassion of his, and in return, many were protective and cared about Blake.

He learned best when there could be a follow through with individual attention. He was intelligent and understood the material. He needed some help to get started on assignments. Follow through was most important as it gave him the confidence and encouragement to complete his task. There were many times when we would revisit lessons as there may have been a distraction at lesson time that consumed him or caused him to lose focus.

Group activity sessions were daunting, and it was best to keep Blake in a small setting. Any type of confusion or disorganization was stressful and needed to be avoided.

I hold cherished memories from my year with Blake in Grade 1. He was a wonderful boy, kind, sensitive, intelligent, interesting and fun. Our class was a better place with him in it. Blake taught us as much as we taught him.

In elementary school, my safe person was Robin Spry. She was my Grade 4 teacher and then became my special education teacher for the remaining four years. She was my saviour (my mom would say she was their saviour too). Robin told me that when she was first told she was going to have two autistic students in her class she was very nervous and uneasy. She didn't think she was up to the task. When she looked back, she realized how ignorant she was to have those feelings at the news of having me in her class. Robin reported:

From the start, his parents were so helpful to me and tremendous advocates for Blake, and I knew very early on that they were going to be parents that I would be seeing a lot of. I was mighty relieved after our first meeting during the summer before school started. I am not exactly sure what I expected to see when Blake first walked into my class that day, but he definitely didn't fit the image that I had in my head of a person with an obvious disability. There he was...tall, cute, well spoken, mild mannered...just like any other Grade 4 boy.

Over the years, Blake had several fixations...funny road signs, countries and capital cities, *SpongeBob SquarePants*. He had one particular way to manoeuvre around the classroom. He would always walk around the perimeter of the room and always in the same pattern.

Sometimes Blake seemed to be having a conversation in his head, and sometimes he would laugh out loud even though he wasn't speaking with anyone. Early on, he would stim in the schoolyard by skipping along and flapping his hands. I know he worked very hard not to do this in public as he got older because he recognized it wasn't typical behaviour.

Robin shared some insightful tips for future teachers of autistic students:

- Don't be afraid.
- Embrace the opportunity.
- Learn all you can about autism, including strategies and best practices.
- Have a good relationship with the family.
- Ask questions.
- Take courses.
- Be an advocate for your students.

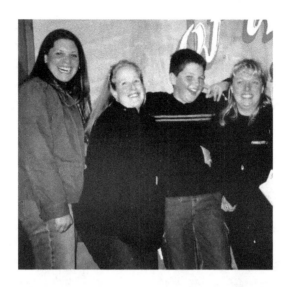

Amazing teaching staff and respite workers I had growing up!

Social Situations, Peer Buddies and Learning to Make Friends at School

A lot of people believe that those on the spectrum prefer to be on their own and not have friends. This may be the case for some, but most of us want friends and have trouble making them. Social situations and making friends was and still is a struggle. Social skills come naturally to *typical* children, but I had to be taught. Sadly, we are often rejected for being different.

I had to be taught that just because one person says "no" or tells me to go away doesn't mean other kids won't want to play with me. There were times when social situations were so tough that I would sometimes say that I didn't want friends, but I really did. I did have friends outside school that I played with at home or at their houses, but somehow it was difficult for me to make friends in the schoolyard. This was most likely because at home I had my parents or an adult close by to help if I needed it, and this was not always the case at recess.

Starting in Grade 1, Vicki Miron, my respite worker, came by at recess and prompted me to ask other students if they wanted to play. She showed me how to do it in a way that I felt comfortable. It was difficult, and I hated having to go outside my comfort zone. Sometimes I would be frustrated because I wanted to have friends to play with but nothing seemed to be working. It seemed like no matter what I did I just could not play and socialize on the playground like the others. I often just wanted to give up, but I knew that my parents would never allow that. They kept pushing me to be social.

Mar 25, 03

gr 3

Arrived at school today to find Blake standing next to the school.
I asked him what he is suppose to be doing and he replied "Today is Tues, you don't usually come on Tues."
I asked what are you suppose to do at lunch when I'm not here. He admitted grudgedly PLAY.

He went back in for a ball & asked Jessica to play. He invited Cole as well and things seem to go well

Vicky

Note to my mom about me not playing at recess like I was supposed to

It wasn't until Grade 3 that I began to feel more comfortable on the playground and schoolyard. That same year, my special education teacher started a Peer Buddies program. The program ran on a schedule, and volunteer students would be assigned to play with me on certain days. This seemed to help, and after some training most of them had a better understanding of me, but I still felt a little nervous asking others to play or hang out. The thing is, children should not have to be told to play with someone who is autistic and is alone on the playground;

they should just do it naturally. I wish that kids had asked me to play without being told to.

With the Peer Buddies, we would do things like play sports, have conversations and do indoor activities when we couldn't go outside. By Grade 5, I started to enjoy having these Peer Buddies, and being in social situations rarely felt like a chore. I recall getting upset when one of the kickball players seemed to be breaking the rules of the game and I expressed my anger to this person with words. I later found out that this kid wasn't breaking the rules on purpose; he had just never played before. This was when the Peer Buddies taught me that when someone breaks the rules of a game it's not always on purpose or to be mean.

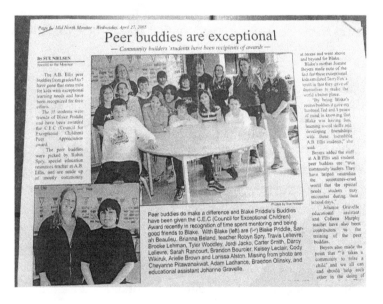

Peer Buddies featured in local newspaper for exceptional efforts

Even though my social skills were improving, I still needed prompting by my educational assistant (EA) on occasion, and an award system was put in place for when I did something social or played without being asked. One day I decided I didn't need the award system anymore because I felt that having Peer Buddies had helped me make friends. That was better than any award I might get.

The Peer Buddies program wasn't all about me. It also helped other kids who had autism or social difficulties. Sometimes I would step in and tell them the things I knew about autism, and this made me feel like I was part of the group.

By the time I reached my pre-teens, I had the social skills necessary to hang out with kids my own age, and I felt a lot more comfortable approaching people. I thank my parents, teachers, life coaches, EAs and friends for having the courage to push me outside my comfort zone; otherwise, I would not have learned to socialize properly.

Social Stuff to Be Taught Explicitly

My parents told me that learning social skills was more important than any other topic at school. This is what my mom had to say about what it was like to teach me social stuff. I had to be explicitly taught how to act in each situation:

> We didn't care if he couldn't do trigonometry, but he needed to know how to get along with others. From learning age-appropriate greetings to taking turns in a conversation, the list of goals to master took many resources (years and cash!). Blake did not have formalized therapy involving Intensive Behavioural Intervention (IBI) or Applied Behavioural Analysis (ABA). This book is not a manifesto on the pros and cons of any therapy. Rather, we tried lots of different strategies to expose Blake to the social world. By trial and error, we (including Blake) figured out what worked best for him.

Conversational Skills:	Friendships:	Self-Awareness:
- Start, join, maintain, end conversation - Shift topics - How and when to interrupt - Ask when don't understand - Say "I don't know" - Complimenting - Orient toward person - Follow multiple step instruction	- Understand what makes true friend - Respect personal boundaries - Detect level of interest from others - Deal with peer pressure - Get attention in positive ways - Understand teachers enforce rules (not you) - Apologize when needed	- Recognize own feelings - Use self-monitoring strategies - Respond appropriately to others emotions - Ask for help - Deal with mistakes - Try when work is hard - Accept praise - Use positive self-talk - Stay calm when stressed
Social Play:	**Conflict Management:**	**Perspective Taking:**
- Turn taking - Compromising - Deal with win/lose - Initiate/sustain play	- Give and accept criticism and deals with bullying in positive ways - Agree to disagree	- Identify and react to feelings and emotions in others and self - Offer comfort

Look at all the social skills to master

Since Blake was verbal, he worked on honing conversation skills. Who knew there were thousands of mini-skills to teach and learn in order to master this social world?

Social scripts were a big part of how Blake learned to converse. With his strength of echolalia, he could repeat almost everything (that he wanted to repeat, that is!). Therefore, we used videos and role modelling to show him the ways to connect verbally with others. It was hard work for everyone, including Blake. Once he mastered one step, we would add another part, mix it up with someone else and work toward generalization. We did this slowly and methodically over the years.

I can't imagine the incredible mental energy and effort he had to muster 24/7 to figure out this complex social world of ours.

Social Stories were a common thing I was taught to use after I had misread a social situation, needed to better understand what went down and to learn how to act in the future. I wrote hundreds of Social Stories over the years and they were very helpful. Here is what makes up the four parts to a Social Story:

> **Descriptive:** These sentences state where a situation occurs, who is involved, what they are doing and why.

> **Perspective:** These sentences describe feelings and reactions of others in the situation.

> **Directive:** These sentences state what the child is expected to do or say.

> **Control:** These sentences help develop strategies so the child can remember what to do next time. They help the child understand the situation and incorporate past experiences or special interests to help remember and generalize.

For example, here's a Social Story that explains why I was disruptive in the school lunchtime lineup:

The bell goes at lunchtime (descriptive).
The kids usually eat in the lunchroom (perspective).
The kids know the bell tells them it's time to line up (perspective).
We have a line-up to be fair to those kids who wait the longest (perspective).
As each kid gets to the line, they go to the end (directive).
When you arrive, you will try to join the end of the line too (directive).
It's good to try and stand quietly until your turn (directive).
Lunch lines and turtles are both slow (control).
Sometimes they go, sometimes they stop (control).
My teacher will be pleased I have waited so patiently (perspective).
This story can be changed at any time. (This last sentence ends each Social Story to make me think more flexibly).

To increase my ability to accept changes in routine, they often incorporated the words "try," "probably," and "sometimes." My school journals were filled with Social Stories.

My mom told me that in Grade 3, one of the education learning goals listed in my Individualized Education Plan (IEP) was to generate two Social Stories a day. "Virtually every new situation became a Social Story," she said. "Recess and classroom miscommunications were immediately turned into Social Stories. A few of the topics included learning new information, accepting help, how to play games, and what to do when I don't know what to do."

As if putting in lots of hard work learning social skills wasn't enough, I then had to learn to "use" them! One time when I was about eight years old and meeting my mom at her office, her colleague/boss and dear friend, Louise, remembered our interaction:

> I clearly recall one day when Blake was with his mom, and he dropped into my office to say hello. Blake held out his hand for a powerful handshake, and then his mom prompted him to look me in the eyes. I realized then and appreciate even more now how much daily rituals like greetings and social conversation were hard work and required commitment and courage. From a young age, Blake was also very good at asking questions, and it is pretty amazing where this has taken him in his career.

This Language Stuff is Hard—for Everyone!

Being autistic and a literal thinker means I get the intended meaning of a conversation or situation wrong about 90% of the time. In school, this led to many reactions. The teacher might yell at me or tell me I'm wrong, one of my classmates might eye-roll or I could be ignored.

My mom helped teach my peers in the Peer Buddies program some things about social communication. Below is a cool exercise adapted from Andrew Matthews' book *Making Friends* (1990, p.129) we did in Grade 5 to show how easy it is to get the wrong meaning if the tone is on a certain word. *Typical* kids naturally learn the nuances that come with tone, inflection or emphasis on certain words when listening to the speech of another person. I did not learn this easily. These subtle cues tell us the intended meaning of the sentence. I still have some trouble with this, but I am better equipped to ask for clarification now.

Have a go at this sentence which seems straightforward:

I didn't say she broke my pencil can mean up to eight different things depending on which word is emphasized!

I didn't say she broke my pencil [but *someone* said it].

I *didn't* say she broke my pencil [I *definitely* didn't say it].

I didn't *say* she broke my pencil [but I *implied* it].

I didn't say *she* broke my pencil [but *someone* broke it].

I didn't say she *broke* my pencil [but she did *something* with it].

I didn't say she broke *my* pencil [she broke *someone else's*].

I didn't say she broke my *pencil* [she broke *something else*].

Eight of my peers stood in front of the class and each read one sentence emphasizing their specific word. Then the rest of the class described what each sentence meant. My mom said it was a terrific eye-opener for everyone. What they also learned was to ask their autistic peer for clarification before rejecting them by asking, "Blake, do you mean…," or "This is what I mean…."

What Worked for Us: Language Understanding

When my mom wasn't trying to show people at the school how to improve my social communication skills, she was passing on tips to my family. Here's an excerpt from her journal when I was about six years old:

Rarely was Blake not working on his communication skills. One summer, he stayed at the family camp with his cousins and aunt and uncle. What follows is a list of tips I gave my brother and sister-in-law to guide them when interacting with Blake. I'm not sure they knew what they were getting into.

- Get his full attention before speaking: "Blake, I want to tell you…"
- Speak slowly.
- Repeat and re-phrase important messages. If it appears he doesn't understand, especially if he responds inappropriately, that's a good sign he doesn't understand what you said, therefore say it slightly differently.
- After repeat/re-phrasing something, also ask questions to make sure he has processed it. "In two minutes, put your toys away. Make sure you put your toys away in two minutes. When do you have to put the toys away?"
- Pause between thoughts to allow time for him to process the idea. "After dinner, I'd like you to colour…you can watch TV after you finish colouring…just make sure you're ready for bed by eight o'clock."
- Keep your sentences short. If you're upset with him, say, "I'm very upset with you right now…I'm mad because…." NOT: "You know every time I tell you to do something it seems blah blah blah…."
- Encourage him to ask questions when he doesn't understand. Let him know that asking questions shows a person is listening well and cares enough to understand what he is saying. Get him to say, "I don't understand" or "I don't know," rather than something tangential, inappropriately off-topic/jargon.
- Explain idioms or other figurative language. "He's feeling under the weather" means "He's not feeling well."
- Ask specific questions, not open-ended ones. "Did you see Nick score a goal?" not "Tell me about the baseball game."

- After watching movies or videos, help him to reconstruct the story in sequence. Draw pictures of important scenes and put them together in order. Print captions under them.
- Use new words over and over in many different contexts.
- Offer choices when trying to elicit descriptive language: "Blake, does that pineapple taste sweet or sour?"
- Play games where you describe things you see as you drive, and use as many words as possible. For example, tall, striped, soft, funny.
- Help him learn categories and the words that belong in them. For example, furniture, jewelry, fruits.
- Correct time sequences. When he says "yesterday" and means last summer, say "Oh yes, last summer you did…."

You Literals Kill Me

A lot of people on the spectrum take things literally, and I was no different. When I say "take things literally," I am talking about popular idioms and sayings. One of my earliest memories was when I was three years old. I was holding a balloon when I accidentally let go and it flew away. I was really upset that I lost it, and Mom tried to comfort me by saying that the balloon was going to fly to McKerrow, the place where we lived. After she told me that, every time I saw a balloon flying away, I thought it was going to McKerrow.

One time I was with Cam, my brother from another mother, at Vicki's house. Now Cam was a bit of a rascal and loved playing tricks and being silly. To tease me he would say, "I'm going to get you." I didn't have the words to tell him I didn't like that. One day after telling me he was going to get me, he picked me up. I was so afraid I bit his arm. We both laugh at this incident now, and Cam told me he didn't know I was different back then. Had he known I didn't understand he would never have used that phrase.

My Grade 1 teacher, Cathy Clackett, recalled that I didn't always understand teasing from my classmates either:

Blake would read and process comments by others in a different way. I tried to be cognizant and help him interpret these statements. Various social interactions were problematic often because of a misunderstanding in the verbal statements.

On one occasion, Blake ran into the classroom after recess, upset and frantic because someone in the yard had told him that they were going to "kill him." Blake totally believed this individual and he feared for his life! It took a while to calm him down and convince him that the comment was just an expression. It was a funny incident for some, but not for Blake.

He struggled with such comments, but as time went on, he learned the ropes and would laugh with us when he really understood. We loved those times when he found humour in himself and his interpretations.

Some idioms, such as "cut it out," came naturally, but most did not. When I was told it was "raining cats and dogs," I would look out the window to see if there really were cats and dogs falling from the sky. If someone said I had "ants in my pants," I would look down my pants to find them. My speech therapist started teaching me the meanings of these sayings. The first one was "elbow grease," which I thought was something you put on your elbows, not hard work. I also learned some idioms that my peers had never heard before like "You're full of hot air," "Not my cup of tea," or "Go fly a kite." It felt good to know I learned something my classmates did not know.

I felt better about taking things literally after seeing a sketch on one of my favourite shows, *The Amanda Show* called "The Literals." This episode was about a family that took everything—and I mean everything—literally. The first time I saw that sketch I said to myself, *Maybe I am not so "out to lunch" after all.*

One of my best family friends, Eliza, remembered me taking Dad's comment literally at New Years:

We were eating dinner, and Ted made some comment along the lines of "It's New Years, you can do whatever you want!" Blake interpreted this literally and took the opportunity to squeeze the juice from a lime over my head. I was about twelve at the time, so I didn't think it was very funny (I was a pouty, moody pre-teen, sorry), but now I think it's hilarious!

If you have a child on the spectrum who takes things literally, introduce them to a new idiom or figure of speech at least once a week and ask them what they think the idiom means. If they don't know, you can tell them the meaning in a way they will understand and use the idiom in a sentence. Once you think they know enough about idioms, have them look for one you have never heard of in a book or on the internet. Be creative and have fun with it.

My parents have lots of funny and not-so-funny examples of teaching me to think "outside the box"—beyond black and white, literal thinking. What follows is a story from my mom that shows my flexible thinking was still a work in progress:

Ice cream. Everyone in our family LOVES ice cream. As a dietitian, I don't promote using food as a reward, but I have to say there are exceptions to healthy eating guidelines. Raising kids is difficult. Once you figure out what motivates your kid, I say go for it. So, I call it an incentive, not a bribe.

When Blake was about seven or eight years old, I would pick him up from school a few days a week and we would go to Tony's Convenience Store for an ice cream cone. It was a month's long lesson broken into myriad steps to teach Blake how to order and pay for his own cone. Seems like a simple, easy thing to learn—until you have a literal learner.

Blake mastered getting out of the car, watching both ways to cross the street safely and entering the store. Then he had to read the situation: where does the unmarked line-up start? When to order. Paying attention to the clerk who mumbles, giving the right amount of money, not getting ripped off with change owed and remembering to be polite with appropriate pleasantries when the transaction was complete. Then leaving the store, crossing the road and getting back into the car where I waited.

After several modelling practises, it was "go on my own" day for Blake, so I parked across from Tony's. Blake jumped out of the car and waited for the traffic to pass. Okay, there's a car one kilometre away but since he can see it, he doesn't cross. First literal interpretation.

As he waits to cross the street, four kids pile into the store. Instantly, I worry. *What if they bug him? Stop it, Jo.* I see a police cruiser pull up in front of Tony's. *Oh good, those kids won't bug Blake with a cop in the store,* I think to myself.

Four kids emerge by the time Blake enters. Then I wait. And wait. And wait. What could possibly be taking so long? *Calm down, Jo.*

Five minutes later, Blake exits Tony's, looks both ways, crosses safely and hops in the car—without an ice cream cone.

"Hey honey, where's your cone?"

"I didn't have enough money, Mom."

After several minutes of piecing it all together, apparently Blake wanted two scoops (we had practised ordering only one!), and when he went to pay, he was short fifty cents. The police officer waiting in line at the counter offered to pay the difference but Blake said, "No thank you. My parents told me never to accept money from strangers."

Black and White Thinking

Thinking in black and white almost always involves needing to have things a certain way. If things are different than the person expected or wanted, it could cause them to become upset. Taking a different route home, being served different looking food or stretching rules—things that don't bother others—can really bother an autistic person. We tend to think in black and white because when something is different than what we expect it can cause confusion, mixed messages and panic.

In kindergarten, Jami remembered an incident at school that left her mom (Vicki) and me in tears. She recalled:

When Blake got something in his little mind, that was it. I remember coming home from school one day to find my mom was mad and Blake was upset. My mom told me that when Blake got off the bus he was upset because his teacher had told him he didn't have any brothers or sisters. Technically, he doesn't, but because he spent so much time at our house and we loved him SO much, Blake considered us his brothers and sisters, just as we thought of him as a little brother...from another mother.

Anyway, his teacher had said to the class, "Whoever has brothers or sisters can go get dressed for the bus." Since we lived in small-town Espanola, Blake's teacher knew that he did not have any brothers or sisters and that our family babysat him. His teacher could have allowed him to get dressed for the bus and not cause him unnecessary upset. Instead, the teacher insisted that Blake did not have brothers or sisters and did not allow him to get dressed for the bus. This was very upsetting for him, and understandably so.

When Blake got off the bus and my mom found out why, she grabbed the photo calendar and was ready to go back to school to explain to the teacher that he did, in fact, have brothers and sisters even if they came from different parents! Every year at Christmas, Blake's mom would make a photo calendar with pictures of Blake and the Adams family. This was a great example of his extended family. I am sure Vicki set that teacher straight. My mom treated Blake like one of her own and loved him just as much.

When I was about seven years old, we went to visit Grandma Dot in Florida. One day we went to a restaurant for "brunch," which my parents told me was like having breakfast and lunch together. Because of that, I thought I needed to have some breakfast food and lunch food at the same time. At first, my mom and dad refused to allow me to do this. Rather than end up with a meltdown, they decided to let me have both breakfast and lunch, literally. I ordered scrambled eggs and toast and then I had a burger and fries. A typical person would simply order one meal and call that brunch, but it took me a while to understand that brunch doesn't mean you literally have to eat two meals. I did manage to eat everything on both my plates that day, and I even had an ice cream sundae afterward! It's little things like this in life that make wonderful and happy memories that we can all look back at and laugh.

Food was a big part of my black and white thinking, especially French fries. Whenever I went to a restaurant, I always needed to have fries with a meal. My parents would not allow me to eat fries twice in the same day or even the day after eating fries because, as most of us know, eating them all the time isn't good for you. However, I thought they were good for me since they are vegetables. If I didn't have fries with a meal my mind could not let it go and I would feel overwhelmed with stress. Sometimes I would have a complete meltdown and other times my parents would give me the option of having fries again instead of dessert. Having this option helped ease the anxiety brought on by my black and white thinking. One time Mom and Dad said "no" to French fries, but they didn't say anything about onion rings so I ordered those instead! That is when I learned deep fried foods are not to be eaten every day.

As I grew older, I began to understand why it's not a good idea to have fries all the time, and I felt more comfortable ordering rice or a baked potato or mashed potatoes as a side dish instead. I commend my parents for trying to make me eat healthy, although it hasn't fully worked as I probably eat worse now as a grown-up than I did then (sorry Mom!).

Despite the negative effects of thinking in black and white, it had benefits as well. There is an old saying that "Rules are meant to be broken." Not for me. The thought of breaking any rules, however minor, was enough to make me feel anxious. As a result, I listened to my parents 99.9% of the time because of my strong conscience.

It is also fairly common for autistics to go through a phase of being "the rules police." I was no exception, although I wasn't aware I was being that way. My mom found an excerpt in my Daily Communication Book from my Grade 2 teacher where I ratted out a boy who apparently was rude to another kid. Since I understood that things like hitting, stealing, talking back to the teacher and skipping school were not allowed, I would do whatever I could to ensure I didn't break these rules because I knew I would get in trouble. But knowing that I broke a rule felt even worse than being punished.

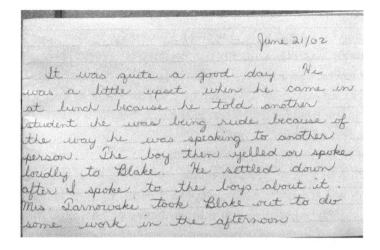

June 21/02

It was quite a good day. He was a little upset when he came in at lunch because he told another student he was being rude because of the way he was speaking to another person. The boy then yelled or spoke loudly to Blake. He settled down after I spoke to the boys about it. Mrs. Larnowski took Blake out to do some work in the afternoon.

In Grade 2, I was practising being the *rule police*

Even when adults told me it was okay to stretch some rules, I had a hard time. One time, my mom's friend Lanny told us that her daughter Grace was hell bent on staying up until midnight on New Year's Eve. Because Grace was only four years old, Lanny wanted to trick her into thinking that it was midnight when it was really only eight o'clock at night. That way Grace could celebrate and then when she went to bed, we would all stay up. It was unthinkable to me that we would lie to Grace even though I was told over and over that it was okay. I could not wrap my head around the fact that two adults whom I looked up to and had taught me that playing tricks on people was wrong suddenly wanted me to play a trick on a four-year-old girl. I felt so confused and anxious. Over the years I did learn how to stretch and break minor rules, but it didn't happen overnight.

This is just my black and white thinking in a nutshell. It continued well into my teen years, and I still think this way to this day.

Dealing with Unexpected Changes

Dealing with changes and inconsistencies was very difficult for me. I felt silly that I wasn't able to handle changes as easily as typical kids. Now I understand that it's nothing to be embarrassed about. There are ways to handle unexpected changes, since life is full of them, and believe me I have had to deal with all kinds up to today.

A phrase I hated hearing my parents say was "We will play it by ear" because it wasn't an answer. It made me uncomfortable because I didn't know what to expect. Why couldn't we just do things on a set schedule? It took a long time for me to accept the fact that life is unexpected and not run by a schedule.

One of my respite workers and a family friend, Miranda, was going to take me to a movie, but we ended up missing it because we didn't have a movie schedule. That upset me. Before Miranda and I left the theatre, she gave me a chance to calm down. I thank Miranda for having the guts to put me outside my comfort zone and for understanding at the same time.

When I was eleven, I really wanted a girl that I liked to come to my house for a sleepover. I'd had girls sleep over in the past, so I didn't think it was a big deal. Mom and Dad explained (or tried to) that when boys get to the puberty stage it's no longer appropriate to have girls at a sleepover. This really upset me and I fought *tooth and nail* to change their mind because I didn't understand the logic. It had been okay in the past, so why was it suddenly not okay? It wasn't until I got a firm talking to from Dad that I finally accepted this as the way it had to be. "You have to be thankful you are having a birthday party (actually two!), and if you keep up this attitude, you'll have none." These words snapped me out of my mindset and made me realize I was the one being unreasonable. Dad's tough love talks have taught me so much. And, of course, as I got older, I figured out the optics of inviting girls over for sleepovers.

My Aunt Janet remembered initially thinking that all kids are persistent and prefer routine. Once she experienced me first hand, however, she realized that autism took coping with changes to a new level:

> When Blake was about eleven years old, he and his parents visited me in Vancouver. Jo warned me that Blake was quite obsessive about whales, but I thought it wouldn't be a problem because my son used to become obsessed with things so I was used to it. Jo said, "No,

you will see this is different," and I saw what she meant as the holiday went on.

Blake had a video about whales that he kept playing over and over until Jo finally said that was enough. He was excited about visiting the aquarium because there were beluga whales there. When we got to Stanley Park I bought two tickets to go on a horse-drawn carriage ride around the park. Blake got into the carriage, but was upset to the point he was shaking and crying because he was so determined to see the whales first. Jo calmed him down and we had a pleasant carriage ride through the park. After we went to the aquarium, Blake was in heaven.

A few days into our visit I said to Jo, "You are right, this is not the same as my son."

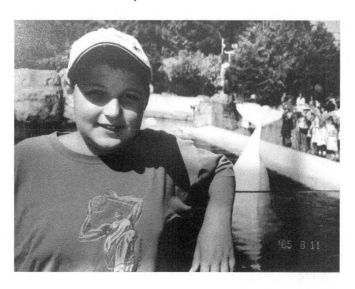

Getting to see the beluga whales at the Vancouver Aquarium

The summer I was thirteen was no picnic for many reasons. I tried to wean off my anxiety medication, I had a math tutor, and I had a painful dental appliance inserted into my mouth. On top of all that, my parents constantly changed our vacation plans. One day we were going camping at Lake Superior, my favourite place to go, then they'd cancel and we stayed at the family cottage instead. Lots of plans changed that summer. It was my first real taste of learning to be flexible. Many a meltdown occurred that summer.

Fortunately, I still had a good summer even though everything was unpredictable. I was put back on my meds later that year, which helped me manage my anxiety better. I guess without having all of these experiences I would never have learnt how to deal with changes I am faced with as an adult. Nowadays, I try to go with the flow as much as I can, and I am glad my parents were not afraid to expose me to life's many changes. If people on the spectrum have these kinds of experiences, they stand a better chance of being able to handle changes. I no longer hate the words "play it by ear," and I try to embrace them because sometimes good things come from things that are least expected.

The Fire Drill: Irrational or Rational Fear?

For as long as I can remember, I had a big fear of the fire alarm at school. It wasn't until Grade 4 or 5 that I had the courage to admit my fears because I was afraid of being made fun of. To try to help me overcome this fear, I was allowed to wait outside and watch as the principal or the custodian pulled the alarm for a fire drill. The teachers would also tell me about it ahead of time to prepare me for the loud noise. This helped, but if it was up to me, I would rather have waited outside every time the fire alarm was pulled. They couldn't let me do that because I needed to know what to do if there really was a fire.

My mom tried to put me outside my comfort zone and make me go through with a fire drill without waiting outside, and I felt as if she was forcing me to jump off a cliff. We had a big argument over it. But if she hadn't done it, I may never gotten over my fear of fire alarms. Now I can handle the noise like a pro.

Here's my mom's take on how I handled fire alarms:

The fire drill played a looming role in Blake's life throughout school (and in any public building for that matter. The time the alarm went off when he was in the public indoor pool meant no swimming for months afterward).

In retrospect, I probably should have been more tolerant of this fear. I wish I'd known more about hypersensitivity and how unique and finely tuned Blake's sensory abilities are. I should have been more accepting that his fear of the fire drill was legit. I imagine it was startling for a few reasons. Firstly, the noise was unexpected, so anticipating it brought on paralysis for hours or days before the alarm was set off. Secondly, it was obnoxiously LOUD, more so because he has super power hearing.

In his seventh year of elementary school, the anticipated fire drill still figured predominantly as a recurring theme in his Daily Communication Book.

> **EA:** Fire drills this week. I didn't tell Blake. I wasn't sure if he was going to fixate about it. I was going to warn him tomorrow morning.

> **Jo**: Please DON'T warn him about the drill. When it occurs, reassure him. "Be calm, we will walk outside and wait a few minutes, then go back in."

> NEW PLAN: after thirty minutes of tears and a panic attack at home tonight, the best approach is: warn him five to ten minutes before, and have him accompany you and watch the custodian pull the switch, then go right outside.

EA: The fire drill went excellently. He was very nervous. We met the custodian at the alarm, and he asked Blake if he would like to pull the alarm.

"God, NO!" Blake said.

Haha! Blake had no problems with the evacuation and said he would like to pull the alarm next time. He just doesn't want to get in trouble! We will do a Social Story tomorrow on "When we pull the fire alarm" (only when there is a real fire, never as a prank or when it is for a planned fire drill).

Family Trips Filled with Changing Schedules and Expectations Make Me Flexible!

Living in a big country like Canada often means having to travel long distances just to visit relatives and friends, so I was no stranger to travel during my childhood.

The first time I went on a plane was to visit Grandma Dot in Florida. I had just turned four, and we went to a zoo and an amusement park. I really enjoyed Busch Gardens since I loved animals and I got to see my favourite animals, elephants, for the first time. Going to Disney World and meeting Woody from *Toy Story* was the highlight. My least favourite part was going on Space Mountain. Four-year-old kids aren't allowed on this ride, but my mom figured since I was so tall it would be okay. We had no idea it would be a roller coaster in the dark that went upside down. As soon as the ride started, my mom was scared to death and held on to me for dear life. I had no time to react because I was shell-shocked. Needless to say, my mom felt awful. It was so traumatizing I couldn't face the next ride, It's a Small World After All, which was intended for really little kids.

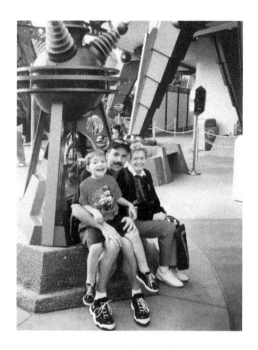

Just finished with Space Mountain—I was pumped!

My first major road trip was from Ontario to Colorado when I was five. I was used to long car trips, so I travelled pretty well. This was before iPads and electronic devices were used to occupy kids on long trips, but, thankfully, I didn't need that since Mom and Dad kept me occupied with books and games. One of my favourite parts of this road trip was seeing prairie dogs in a big field in Nebraska. They were featured on *Zoboomafoo*, my favourite wildlife show. We stopped at a small zoo where there was a capybara, an animal my parents had never seen before. When I told them what it was my dad didn't believe me. He thought it was a made-up word until he looked at the sign that confirmed the name. I think he was embarrassed about being outsmarted by a five-year-old! Not knowing where we would sleep each night taught me flexibility, which was just one of the skills at play in this trip.

We eventually arrived in Boulder, Colorado, where we would stay with our family friends, Leigh and John. I enjoyed staying at their house, but I have to admit I liked the hotels better since they all had pools. Leigh and John are both world travellers and they have inspired me to travel. One day I hope to visit a country they have never visited so I can share my adventures with them.

One of my favourite parts of that trip was when we took the train up Pikes Peak, one of the tallest mountains in the state. Sitting in the last car in the rear seats, my parents were terrified because they felt as if they we were going to fall off the mountain. Since I was a fan of trains, I enjoyed the trip and the scenery.

In the summer of 2001, I got to go camping for the first time at Lake Superior Provincial Park with my mom, her friend Laura and her kids. This trip did not go as planned, but we had some good laughs. The first mistake was forgetting to bring the camp stove, which we needed since there was a fire ban. We were grateful that some fellow campers agreed to lend us their stove. The first night in the tent was not a good one for me since there was a big thunderstorm and we had water dripping in the tent. My first impressions of sleeping in a tent were not good, but my mom and Laura helped me through the night. The next night was better, and I fell asleep to the sound of the waves. Like the other trips, this experience helped me get used to being away from home and sleeping in a new place I wasn't used to.

This would mark one of many trips we took to Lake Superior as a family, and we have great memories of those times.

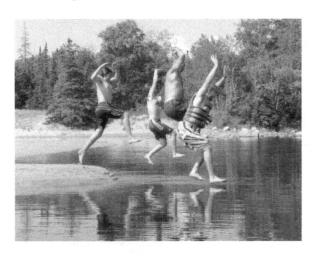

**One of dozens of memories of summers
at Lake Superior Provincial Park**

Anxiety, Fear, OCD and Depression— How Much Can One Person Handle?

"It takes a strong person to admit they need help rather than keeping it a secret."

Me

☆

Anxiety and depression, where do I start with this one? The truth is, all human beings experience these mental states; it's part of being human. Anxiety is a natural emotion, just like fear. It helps keep us safe from danger and serious problems. If we didn't have anxiety, we would all be dead; it is what ultimately kept our ancestors safe from predators. A therapist once told me that our ancestors used fear to escape danger, and we still have a lot of our ancestors' instincts and reactions to danger.

Some people can handle these emotions with no trouble, but others really struggle. The way anxiety feels can differ for each person. Sometimes it feels like having butterflies in my tummy. Other times it feels like I can't calm down and can't breathe to the point where I hyperventilate. And sometimes I feel pain like someone has stabbed me all over my body with a knife. That's the worst kind. It can be unbearable. Panic attacks are also common. If you have never had a panic attack, trust me, you never want to. It literally feels like you are dying.

I have obsessive-compulsive disorder (OCD). My Mom told me it is super common for folks on the spectrum to have what are called "co-morbidities"—other mental-health challenges. Having OCD can bring on a lot of anxiety as well. I am proud of having autism and I would not trade it for the world, but I would gladly trade away my anxiety, depression and OCD.

In elementary school, I had a lot to be anxious about. All kids worry, but I took it to a heightened level where it interfered with how I functioned some days. During grades 3 and 4, natural (tornadoes, earthquakes) and man-made (house fires, plane crashes) disasters bothered me even though I had lots of support and reassurance. In Grade 4, I started to worry about being killed by killer bees or poisonous snakes even though we didn't have them in our region. I don't even want to think about how bad my anxiety would be if the COVID-19 pandemic happened during my childhood; I would never function properly.

Seeing scary things on the news stirred up the anxiety. Even though watching the news may have heightened my anxiety, I was still interested in hearing the stories, and it helped me to learn that sometimes you just can't escape bad news. I am glad my parents let me watch the news at a young age (with supervision).

It was tough to make all these worries go away, but we managed to find something that helped at least for a little while. Before bed, I would tell my worries to one of my miniature worry dolls, and the next morning I would wake up having forgotten what I was worried about in the first place. Worry dolls come from Central America and are said to be magical, but I think my worries went away by talking about them with someone or something.

The anxiety I experienced in my early years was minor compared to what I faced in Grade 5. I started to experience what we used to call my "icky thoughts," a form of intrusive thinking which is a symptom of OCD. This was a huge test of my sanity because I often imagined I had done bad things like start fires or hurt people. In a way it's normal for human beings to have these thoughts as long as we don't act on them. I would never act on these things and that's what's important. The problem was, I was only eleven, and I was trying to figure out fact from fiction. Whenever I had these icky thoughts, I felt like I was a bad person. My parents, therapists and those who cared about me explained that these were just thoughts and not actions. They said having a conscience to tell me right from wrong and to stop me from doing bad things was a good thing; it showed I was a good person. This helped a little, but these icky thoughts bothered me for several months. I had visual triggers that I needed to learn were just that, triggers. I was unable to look at or use things like matches or things that could be used as a weapon because they would trigger my icky thoughts.

My EA at school did her best to help me work through my icky thoughts and anxiety. In my Daily Communication Book, May 2005, she wrote:

> Blake has been taught to shake his head to get the thoughts out, and I recorded a minimum of fifty-six shakes over a three-hour period. Triggers are simple things. For example, tying his shoes led him to believe that the friction of his shoelaces would cause a fire to start. I am helping him take time out to do some relaxation and express his feelings about his thoughts.

To help cope, my parents paid for a psychologist who specialized in cognitive behavioural therapy (CBT). Despite being an eight-hour drive away, I also saw my amazing London-based psychiatrist several times. He helped figure out what I was dealing with and prescribed medication.

My family and I went to Florida for a couple weeks so I would have a change of scenery and work on the CBT strategies I had learned. I still had some anxious episodes, but they weren't as bad as they were back home. I was able to take my mind off the negative voice in my head by going swimming and seeing wildlife. The tropical setting helped me feel better.

After I came home, I still had some issues, and at times it got so bad that I was disrespecting my teachers and EAs because I wasn't thinking straight. But in time, I recognized this and apologized.

One trick was to talk back to my conscience, in my head, rather than telling my parents about these thoughts every time I had one. The trick did not help at all at first. I felt like I couldn't have one of my icky thoughts without telling Mom or Dad. It took a long time to learn how to talk back to my conscience, but now I do it all the time when my mind starts playing tricks on me. I tell the negative voice in my head to go away, and then I go on with my day. If talking to the voice doesn't work after a couple of hours or so, I give my parents a ring and tell them what is bothering me.

Dealing with icky thoughts and having my mind play tricks on me was by far the most difficult anxiety to deal with in my childhood. It was so bad that at times I wasn't able to concentrate in school or do anything fun. I felt guilty, miserable and like a bad person all the time. There were even times when I didn't want to live anymore. I never want to deal with that kind of pain again. I wasn't able to watch any action shows, shows with violence or buildings on fire as they set off my anxiety and I would worry that these things would happen to me.

As part of my OCD, I washed my hands until they were red sometimes because I was afraid of being contaminated, contaminating someone else or making them sick. I was even afraid to touch peanut butter or other peanut products because I was worried I would experience an allergic reaction or I would give someone else one. There was nothing I didn't worry about.

On the advice of my psychiatrist, my meds were doubled to reduce my intrusive thoughts. The anxiety medication worked well, but I overdosed a few times and had to leave school early. I kind of laugh now about getting stoned on these drugs back then, but it could have been dangerous. It felt like I was in a dream-like state and completely zoned out. I passed out at my desk more than once until my meds were regulated.

One time when I was learning how to manage my anxiety with breathing exercises on a CD, it kept skipping. My mom and I were laying down breathing to the sound of the man's voice on the CD. The guy told us to breathe in slowly, so we did. Then we heard him say, "Breathe out...breathe out...breathe out...breathe out...breathe out..." over and over. It was the first time I had laughed in a long time. Dad later joked that if I had breathed out any more, I would have passed out. It just goes to show that even in difficult times there is always a way to find happiness no matter how little it may be.

Summer and Speech Camps: Life Lessons

Experiences at summer camps and day camps differ among children. Some have the best memories while others would never go back if their parents paid them. I have been to several speech therapy day camps, local recreation day camps and some overnight camps. I found that I got along the best at local camps mainly because I knew most of the people and the bullying was minimal. But there were other camps I went to that were far from home.

Speech Therapy Half-Day Camp

The first camp I recall going to was in London, Ontario, when I was six years old, shortly after my autism diagnosis. I learned a lot at this camp. Not only were we taught speech, but we also learned about eye contact and recognizing emotions. The way they taught eye contact was very creative. They had us pick a random item out of a bag. Whoever was holding the item would have to make eye contact with the person next to them and describe the item. The rule of this game was to make eye contact, so if you didn't, you had to try again. This was the first time I understood I was supposed to look at someone when I spoke to them. Prior to that, I would often not even face the person all the while looking at my feet while talking. Making eye contact or at least turning my body towards the person took me a few years to master.

To teach us about feelings, they had us cut out pictures of faces from newspapers and magazines and glue them to paper. We presented our collages to the instructors and described the faces as best we could. Then they asked us how each person was feeling. For instance, if I pointed to a sad face, I would say, "This person is sad because he has a frown on his face." This technique taught me about emotions, but it is a lot more difficult to tell how a person is feeling in real life than it is to describe the emotions in a picture.

The thing I liked about this day camp was that everything was structured and we followed a schedule posted with pictures. I could read at the time, but the pictures helped a lot. I also enjoyed the calm nature of the program and the fact that it was only two hours a day. I felt very relaxed in this environment, but my enjoyment of camp the following summer made it a distant dream.

Camp for Kids with ADHD

The camp I attended the next summer was not fun at all, but it made me a wiser kid. This day camp in London was six hours a day instead of just two. There weren't many leaders, and there were lots of older kids who I thought were intimidating. Also, it was a camp that was targeted toward kids with ADHD, something I did not have.

The first couple of days were okay, but by the third day I started to feel uncomfortable because of the chaos. These kids always had to be doing something active. There was no way they could just sit and do crafts or something quiet, which is what I needed to do to feel more comfortable. Because of all this chaos, I would start crying halfway through the day and it wouldn't stop until my parents picked me up. The counsellors did not really know how to help me when I was in distress, and one counsellor decided to hug me when I was crying, even after I said "no." That was scary because I did not like being hugged without permission, and I certainly didn't like being hugged by people I didn't know.

At the end of the week, I convinced my mom that I did not want to go back. She understood how I felt, so I didn't have to. This camp helped me prepare for situations that are unstructured and unpredictable, and it helped me deal with situations where I would not always have someone whom I knew to help me.

Speech Therapy Full-Day Camp

In 2002, I started my first of two years at a London speech therapy full-day camp called "Talk about Fun" where I would work on some speech goals. Although I had a better time at this camp, I found it difficult to adjust mainly because the staff didn't know me and what I needed to fit in. It was sort of like school but with a really small number of students. I went back to this camp during March Break for half days, which made me feel better, but my mom signed me up for full days in the summer with the option of attending half days if things didn't work out. Having this option made me more comfortable. In time, the workers got to know me and I managed to have a good time.

"Talk about Fun" camp introduced me to the notion that changing topics without giving people notice was confusing for them. I had a tendency to do that, but I learned to say "change of topic" when I wanted to talk about something else. My parents and I still use those three words to this day!

One of my speech goals was to learn about sarcasm—not an easy thing to master! Even today I often ask, "Are you being sarcastic?" when I'm listening to someone to make sure I don't misread the conversation.

Sleepover Summer Camp: First Year FUN, Second Year HELL

Toward the end of the summer, I spent a week at a sleepaway YMCA camp called "John Island" in northern Ontario. My mom contacted an agency that provided one-on-one counsellors for kids like me to attend sleepover camps. My counsellor was well-trained in the first year and knew how to help me if I was having a hard time. What I liked about this camp was taking part in all the cool activities. More importantly, the counsellor didn't tolerate any bullying. This made me feel safe and like I belonged.

The second year at John Island was a nightmare. The counsellor assigned to me did not have a clue about autism. I was constantly bullied and put down by the boys in my cabin for being different, and, unlike the previous year, the counsellor did nothing to stop the bullying. Because of that, I felt that I had to stand up for myself by being mean back to the kids, but that only made it worse. I stuck it out for the week but never went back to overnight summer camp again.

Despite all the problems I had at these camps, attending them was beneficial. I learned that I won't always have someone I trust to go to when something is wrong and that there will always be bullies in the world. So I encourage everyone with children on the spectrum to put their kids in an appropriate camp where there is support. Camps expose them to the real world and are one of the best ways to help them understand others and grow.

Early Memories of Bullying: Sticks and Stones May Break My Bones, but Words Will Never Hurt Me—Said No One EVER!

"Crying doesn't mean you are a coward. The first thing you do when you are born is cry; it's a sign of life and it shows that you are alive. Sometimes it takes a real man to show their emotions."

Me

☆

Thankfully, I didn't have to deal with bullying *every day* in my childhood. But, no matter how good one's life is, there are always going to be cruel people out there. I have learned that people like that mean nothing to me and they are not worth getting upset over. The saying, "Never serve anyone a meal that you would not want to eat yourself" is a good rule to live by. Now, I simply ignore bullies, but like all life skills this was something I had to learn.

The first time I remember being bullied in a school setting was in senior kindergarten. There was a group of kids that used to poke me with their toys almost every day at recess. I didn't know why they did this, but it might have been because I was always alone on the playground. I struggled with telling them to stop or that I didn't like what they were doing. It's hard to tell whether these kids were being bullies intentionally, but I tried to ignore them and pretend it never happened. Sadly, one day I'd had enough of these kids and I ended up fighting back by pushing them away. As a result, we were sent to the office.

This bullying continued into Grade 1 and really got out of hand when the same group of kids started punching me. This time, I thought I needed to fight back so I tried to throw a punch at this kid and missed and hit someone else. I felt horrible because I knew that hitting was wrong. Because I felt remorse for hurting someone else, I didn't care that I lost my TV privileges for the night. In my heart I knew I deserved the punishment, but I just wanted all the bullying to stop. This is when I had the courage to tell my parents exactly what was going on at school.

After that, Mom, Dad and my teacher, Mrs. Clackett, taught me how to deal with bullying in a way that would keep me out of trouble. Dad told me to run away from the bullies as fast as I could and if they came closer, I should tell them really loudly to "BACK OFF!" If that didn't work, I was to tell a teacher or a yard supervisor and they would deal with the bullies appropriately. This seemed to work, and once Mom arranged for certain classmates to play with me at recess, the bullying subsided, but there were still some occasional incidents.

Sometimes I took the concept of using my words too far instead of physically responding. I had to learn that calling people names when they bullied me was not okay and that it is also a form of bullying. Prior to this, I was under the impression that bullying only meant using your fists and that calling bullies names is not "using your words." Another strategy I used was to ignore the bully and not react to what they said. If I ignored the bully, they would give up because there was no point in being mean if I didn't react. This strategy worked most of the time, but sometimes not reacting is easier said than done.

One incident I remember well was somewhat petty compared to things that had happened to me previously. I was in Grade 2 and a kid hit me in the head with some mud. I thought I would get him back by tackling him just like football players do—if they could it then I could too. BIG mistake. The other kid was punished, but I also received my first ever detention. I had to learn that even if someone deserves to have something bad happen to them, it isn't right for me to do it. I was ashamed that I had gotten a detention, but the vice principal called my mom to assure her (and me) that the detention would be my only punishment. He was very understanding and even showed me the room where my detention would be the next day so I would know what to expect.

What might have seemed simple to many kids caused so much anxiety in me. This is what my mom recalled of the "Mud Throwing Incident":

The Detention: Grade 2, April 2002

Got a call from the vice principal (VP). We are on a first name basis, and I'm pretty sure he has me on speed dial.

"Blake's a bit upset; can you reassure him?" he asked.

"Sure, what happened?"

"Blake was standing by a pole waiting for the recess bell when another student pushed him and flung mud in his face. Blake tackled one of them."

(*Way to go Blake*, I said to myself)

The VP handed the phone to Blake, and I said, "Blah, blah, blah...We need to learn to use our words, walk away, tell the closest adult..."—the usual rote phrases parents repeat to their child when they get bullied.

Between sobs, Blake blurted, "Will you and Daddy be mad? Does this mean no TV or video games for a month? Forever? What's a detention? Is it every day forever?"

"No, it's for one lunch hour in the library where the rules are to read a book and no talking," I replied.

Tears welled up—mine and his. I heard my wee boy sniffling and could feel the fear washing over his beautiful, flawless face.

"What's wrong, honey?"

"Can I breathe when I'm there having my detention?" Blake cried.

"Of course you can sweetie."

"Okay, I feel a bit better now, Mom."

Both my parents went easy on me that night, and they reminded me what I was supposed to do when I was being bullied at school. This time it really sank in.

Shortly after this incident I had the courage to tell the person in authority if I was being bullied. I didn't want to be punished anymore, and I wanted to be a good student. One day when I was on the schoolyard, a student was messing around and thought it would be funny to pretend to throw a ball at me. He laughed at me afterward, but I didn't find this kid's joke funny; in fact, I felt threatened by his actions. As much as I wanted to get back at him, I remembered what I was told to do in this situation. Most kids would have gone to an adult on the schoolyard, but I asked if I could go see the vice principal instead because I had developed trust in him after the "Mud Throwing Incident." I went to his office and told him what had happened on the schoolyard. He was very proud of me for doing the right thing, and it marked the first time I was able to deal with a bully without getting into trouble. This was a big accomplishment.

I learned that there are many forms of bullying. There is physically being pushed or fighting, being taunted or having others spread lies about you, and being socially excluded or shunned. It was pretty easy to not fight physically, but it was a lot more difficult to pick up the clues for the other forms of bullying. Also, my parents taught me not be a bystander; if I saw someone being bullied, I was to speak up. This sometimes didn't go as planned if I had misread the situation.

Once the Peer Buddies joined me on the playground, the bullying was not as frequent. Having the tools to deal with bullies helped me in the long run. If your child is being bullied, it might help to ask them what is going on and try to figure out how to solve the problem. If there is one thing I learned, it is that if you are being bullied, telling someone you trust is one of the best ways to make it stop. You can even challenge your child by asking him or her what they think they should do if they are ever in a bullying situation to see what answer they come up with.

No matter what, there will always be bullies in the world, but as long as we spend time with the people in our lives who matter and ignore the ones who don't, life will feel a lot better. Just walk away, or if you are being bullied online just log off because bullies don't matter in life; only people that you care about and love matter.

There are Friends and Then There Are Real Friends

This is what I believe to be a real friend:

A friend likes someone else for who they are and doesn't treat them differently. A friend sticks up for someone when they're being bullied or made fun of. I was lucky to have the Peer Buddies program to help me come out of my shell. If you have a kid who doesn't have learning challenges, encourage them to talk to kids who are all alone on the playground and ask if they want to play. If they do it, I just know it will make their day.

Being a good friend can be summed up in three simple points.

Agree to Disagree: We don't have to have the same views to be good friends. We just need to respect different points of view and not force our beliefs on our friends or others. It's even okay to have debates, but insulting others who have differing views or opinions is not okay. It's the way we treat our friends that matters the most, regardless of what we believe. Even if it's something petty like being a Leafs or a Habs fan.

Respect Your Friends' Feelings: This is simple in a way, but it is something even the best of friends may forget. When someone says something that hurts us, we can call them on it in a polite way and be okay when they do the same to us. We need to listen more than talk. It is not a good idea to pressure a friend into doing something that makes them feel uncomfortable; real friends don't push real friends.

Be Yourself: We shouldn't pretend to be someone we're not to make friends or to fit in. If someone doesn't accept us for who we are, they aren't a true friend anyway.

My lifelong true friend is Jakob. We spent a lot of time together during our childhood and were in the same class all through school. Our moms are good friends, and Vicky was one of my life coaches. We were like brothers in a lot of ways. Sometimes we fought non-stop and other times we were best of friends and stood up for each other if one of us was being bullied.

Jakob told me I used to follow him around lot. He recalled a time when we were seven or eight and Vicky let us go by ourselves to a toy store while she did some shopping at the mall. I started to panic because we didn't have an adult watching us and was afraid something might happen, so I started crying. Jakob had done this many times before and it didn't bother him, but he took me back to Vicky who was in another store. He was not a happy chappy having to take a crying friend back to his mom, and this was one thing he never let me forget. We laugh about it now.

Another time, Jakob and I were playing in his backyard with his new toy bow and arrow. He absolutely loved it more than anything. We were on the tire swing and I almost fell off, so instinctively I grabbed the toy bow string. As I pulled myself up, the string of his new favourite toy bow broke. *Now I've done it*, I thought. Jakob completely lost it. He bawled his eyes out and shouted, "He broke it! I am telling!" I wondered how I was going to convince Vicky that it was an accident and worried about what my parents were going to say. I wasn't punished since it was an accident, and Vicky told me not to worry because Jakob was just upset and we would still be friends. I later found out the toy was purchased at the local dollar store so it's no wonder it broke so easily. As we got older, Jakob and I teased one another over these incidents just for fun. Jakob even says I still owe him $1.25 for the bow.

I could go on and on about all the crazy and memorable times I've had with Jakob and his family. Despite all the fights we got into, he is still one of my best friends because he is a true friend. Nothing will change that.

My mom said that when I was in elementary school, one of the most difficult things I had to figure out was what makes a true friend. I learned that being friendly is not the same as being a true friend. There are people we only say hi to, close friends, casual friends, people we pay to help us, and so on. It got even more complicated with social media using the word "Friends."

Grade 5 First Day: Unintentional Social Exclusion

My mom wrote in her journal about my first day in Grade 5:

> If I had to pick between a root canal or standing in a gymnasium full of 500 kids on the first day of school…

I never understood the reasoning, but Blake's school had the student body and us keen parents all meet in the gym and look for kids' names on the wall where each teacher's name was posted. It was bedlam and a cacophony of shrills and groans. Sensory overload! In fairness, due to persistent parental pressure back in June, Blake already knew his teacher and even who his classmates were, which was so helpful to minimize his anxiety (and ours) about potential bullies. However, Blake had to partake in the gymnasium chaos as teachers rounded up their new charges. A line of gawky, animated peers formed and off they went toward their new room.

I nudged Blake to join the line and off we went, me in his shadow a few steps behind. I didn't realize I was holding my breath, fearful of the newness and uncertainty a new school year—all 194 days—brings. New IEP, new relationship building with the classroom teacher and precious EA (if he is "lucky" enough to have one assigned to the class). My heart skipped a beat when I was jolted back to my own first day school jitters. I remembered that anticipation—awaited it with excitement—hoping some of my best friends would not only be in my class but sit beside me!

Blake's teacher opened the door and thirty plus kids jostled for seats; seats that I saw were paired. Blake plopped down in the middle of the classroom, and the desk joined to his sat empty. As the rest filed in, it was like watching musical chairs in action. Kids switched seats at lightning speed as friends found each other. I was standing at the door, fingers crossed that a nice peer would sit beside Blake. Elise, a gentle soul, slid in next to Blake...she turned in her seat and, in a flash, vaulted out. Blake alone again. I wanted to vomit.

Birthday Parties

You may have heard from many parents of children on the autism spectrum that their kids either hate birthday parties because of all the noise and stimulation or that they never get invited. Some people assume that autistics don't want to be invited. This is far from the truth for me and many other people on the spectrum. I used to look forward to my birthday and planning the party. Sometimes I would have it at home or at the bowling alley in town with a bunch of friends.

Once I was invited to a girl's sleepover birthday party when I was ten. It started off fine, but I quickly realized that in some cases girls and boys do different things at a sleepover. This party was really disorganized. We rented a horror movie that the girls insisted on watching. Before the movie had even started, they stopped watching it out of fear that they would be scared or have nightmares. This upset me because I thought it would be cool to see a horror film. I was not as afraid of things as other people because I knew movies were fake. Because I was so upset, I had to take a "time out" from the party, and the older brother played chess with me while the girls were upstairs playing. It helped a little, but I had a sense that things were about to get worse.

When it was finally time to go to bed, I was tired, and the thought of staying up all night was scary for me. As I was getting ready to fall asleep some of the girls started giggling, talking and laughing while I was trying to sleep. This was not normal for me because boys never did things like that when we had sleepovers. Because I was already tired from the chaos of the day, I yelled at them twice to go to sleep, but it didn't work. I was so upset that I had a meltdown in front of the girls. They did not know why I was so upset, but my friend's mom calmed me down and told the girls to be quiet so we could all go to sleep.

I was even more agitated the next day, and I ended up calling one of the girls a bad name. When that happened, everyone thought I was a mean person. One person even said that I "used to be" the nicest person in the class. Hearing that was heartbreaking because I knew I was a nice person who cared about people, and I didn't understand why I had acted that way.

Going home from the party felt good because I'd had enough. To ensure that I would know how to deal with a situation like this the next time, my mom and I wrote another Social Story in my journal. In the end, the girls at the party understood why I behaved the way I did, and they forgave me.

One of those girls, Maureen, recalled our school-aged friendship:

> I noticed Blake was a sensitive guy right away. I noticed how his mom and dad had a certain way of speaking with him that worked most of the time. A lot of the time teachers would upset him by saying things in the wrong tone. I noticed he was so very smart and intuitive. He had his own way of doing things, and I know it was sometimes overwhelming having to do something another way. I found I just had to find ways to speak to him so we could be on the same level of conversation. Most of the time I couldn't keep up with his topics and information because he was so knowledgeable! Blake never cared about petty drama because he was just so fascinated with life!
>
> Unusual traits or habits I noticed would sometimes show up when he was feeling anxious or in a situation that made him uncomfortable. Blake was really good at keeping his cool, but a few times something very small (in our eyes) would happen and it would upset him because any change was a big deal for him.
>
> I think the first time I went to Blake's house was difficult for both of us. It was his space, and he was new to sharing things and cohabiting for a few hours with a friend. I can't remember any bad memories, but there were times Blake would be upset. His parents always assured me it wasn't my fault. I always watched his parents to learn how they spoke to him, their mannerisms, tone of voice and body language because it gave me a sense of how

I should interact with Blake. Being at his house was amazing—so much room to play inside and outside! Blake's parents gave him such a great life.

If you know someone with autism, it is worthwhile to invite them to a birthday party because they may want to take part. If things get to be too much, offer a quiet room so they can calm down and then they can go back to the party when they are feeling better.

Break a Leg!

**"Theatre and radio is more than just acting
or talking into a microphone;
it makes me feel human."**

Me

☆

As far back as I remember I have had a strong interest in theatre and the performing arts. The first time I saw a stage show was a school Christmas concert when I was three. I was drawn to it right away and was upset when I couldn't perform with the actors onstage. This was one of the reasons I was eager to go to school, but I was disappointed when I found out the kindergarten kids did not perform in the Christmas concert. To appease me, they allowed me to sing a few songs onstage before school one day in front of a small audience of my babysitter and a few others. Singing in front of a crowd felt good; it felt like I was being listened to, and it brought me out of my shell. After that, I really hoped I could perform in front of an even bigger audience.

My chance came in Grade 1 when I was in my first Christmas concert. I was one of the tallest, so I was on the top riser. We read a few poems and then sang a song. We had to speak loudly since we didn't have microphones but that didn't bother me because I already had a loud voice! Also, the stage was the one place where I could speak up without being told to use my "inside voice" or to keep my voice down. This helped me in future theatre productions and Christmas concerts.

After seeing a local Young Company play by the Espanola Little Theatre, I immediately wanted to join. My chance came in Grade 6 when Espanola Little Theatre's Young Company was planning a production of *Let's Do Munsch*, a play about Robert Munsch stories. For the audition, I recited *Dr. Seuss's ABC* book in the most dramatic way possible. Dr. Seuss books can be hard to recite sometimes because of all the rhyming and tongue twisters, but I managed it well and had fun. I later learned that one of the most important parts of theatre is having fun onstage because if you're not enjoying yourself then the audience won't enjoy it either.

Sharon and Bob Sproule, both of whom were talented local actors who took a "no nonsense" approach to the project, mentored us during the production. Sharon's style of discipline was somewhat intimidating. For example, if she saw us shaking our legs up and down or flapping our hands onstage, she would notice. It was like she had eyes in the back of her head! She would make us start from the beginning if we did this. She would also threaten to cut off our sleeves or our hair if she saw us playing with them. Keep in mind, she never actually cut off anyone's sleeves or hair, but it was a threat we all took very seriously. Some kids could handle her approach while others could not. It was difficult for me at first, and at times I felt like I had bitten off more than I could chew, but I really wanted to be in a play so I did everything in my power to overcome these obstacles.

Alongside rehearsing for the play, we did other exercises like trying to remember everyone's name. I have a memory like a steel trap, but even that was difficult! One exercise we did really made me feel like I belonged in theatre. We all stood in a work circle, stamped our feet and shouted, "I belong here!" at the top of our lungs. Doing this really made me feel a part of the show, and it also helped me develop a tolerance for loud noises (this play involved a lot of shouting). Some kids needed projection training, but I already had a loud voice and Sharon would later use my voice as a tool for others. She said my voice was "naturally projected."

Despite being a little nervous, our troupe did five flawless performances over four days. Maybe I felt at home onstage because everything was in a script so I knew exactly what to do. The first year of theatre went very well despite the odd bumps in the road. My grandparents and cousins even came to watch me act for the first time. When a play ends it feels a little like a death because the actors are so emotionally connected to it and their colleagues, and this cast was no exception. We ate cake and pizza at the wrap party and shared a few tears, but it felt good to have accomplished something big. Not only did I meet new friends, but I also learned new skills.

Theatre helped me come out of my shell and be more social. My mentor and lifelong friend Sharon Sproule gave her input on my time in theatre:

> The thing that stands out the most for me when I think of the young Blake is the extraordinary understanding and support his mom offered. I'm not sure what prompted Blake to come out to the Youth Theatre when he was twelve, but his mom provided a mentor to be there just for Blake and his "safety." If he had a meltdown, she was there to take him home. I think that because she was there, Blake had that sense of safety that helped so much to make him a functioning member of the group. As he learned to trust me, he quickly fit in and very soon became comfortable enough so that the support worker no longer needed to be there.
>
> I learned so much from Blake!! I didn't realize there were different levels of autism. I was really surprised to find that he didn't know what body language was and that he couldn't read it. I admired his honesty and sense of truth, his strong work ethic, commitment and dedication so much.
>
> Blake's understanding of autism and his openness have had a positive effect on the rest of the theatre companies

with which he has worked. Blake helps them understand and accept people who may have differences and needs other than their own.

I am so grateful for his friendship and loyalty.

I went on to perform in a few more productions with Sharon Sproule, and I learned to recognize certain emotions that people felt through facial expressions and body language. Rather than sitting through boring therapy sessions, I learned these the fun way, through theatre.

Matthew Laurenti, a family friend and local theatre volunteer, remembered an incident involving me:

> I saw two students in the group picking on a young fellow (Blake). They were calling him weird and making fun of the way he walked. I remember thinking to myself how mature Blake was in that situation. He walked away from the bullies with a curious look on his face, deep in thought. I am sure he had composed a way of communicating back to them because he returned to them shortly after and explained that he had autism. He asked them why they would tease him about something he could not control. Blake's ability to communicate his emotions and educate on autism was inspiring and lovely to watch.
>
> Blake has taught me a lot about my own methods of communication, as I am now a nurse. I learned how to treat others with respect and dignity, and that sarcasm isn't universal and can be difficult to understand.

Theatre also taught me to stay focused. I was always focused on the scene when I performed, and I ignored distractions that I would have normally turned to before. Sharon knew right away if we were distracted and made us start over during rehearsal. This was beneficial in the long run, as it helped me to pay attention better in school. Sharon once told us about a time when a play was being performed and a man in the audience had a heart attack. When the paramedics came in and put him on the gurney, everyone in the audience was focused on the man in need of first aid. Meanwhile, the actors continued to act throughout the whole incident. That's the power of theatre.

During the last production with Sharon, one of the actors was not able to handle her strict style. This individual's mother felt that her child was being pushed too hard and even bullied by Sharon. She said some nasty things about her and walked out the door. I was livid. I stood up and said in my biggest voice ever, "What I just heard was absolutely appalling. Sharon you are an amazing person! Before I met you and went into theatre, I was a lonely kid on the playground, literally trapped in my own world. You helped me to find my way out. Without your strict discipline, I might not be where I am today." I burst into tears afterward, and Sharon thanked me.

I truly believe that without Sharon's influence, I would have been too shy to get a job or too afraid to make friends. I owe so much to Sharon, and I am very blessed to have her in my life.

If your child with autism has social anxiety or does not recognize body language or other things that come naturally to typical kids, I recommend enrolling them in theatre. It is a fun and sometimes free way of approaching these challenges. After hearing my success story with theatre, my life coach, Theresa, started a program called "Edge of the Box" that helped kids and teenagers on the spectrum and those with other disabilities to learn social skills, deal with unexpected changes, noises, and other important life skills. The program was successful, as it helped others to come out of their shell. It also gave overworked parents of children with autism a chance to take a break and socialize.

I encourage all parents of autistic children to have their kids do something in the way of performing. You don't have to sign up for an organized drama club or play. You can do it at home; you can make puppets and put on a play, do improvisation, play charades, sing songs or act out scenes from a favourite movie. While you do this, be sure to teach them about feelings and body language as well. If you are creative, the possibilities are endless.

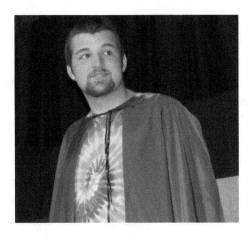

Me in costume for the theatre production
The Seussification of Romeo and Juliet

Pass it to Me!

"Trying new things and going out on a limb is what you have to do sometimes to find out exactly who you are as a person. You won't always find that in the comfort of your basement."

Me

☆

I took part in a wide variety of sports and organized activities in my childhood. I wasn't as interested in sports as many other children were; I liked it, but other times I felt like it was a chore and my parents had to drag me to the sports. Sometimes I felt like saying, "Did it ever occur to you that sports aren't my thing?" But inside, I did want to be like everyone else and play sports. So, I knew I needed to put my best foot forward and try something new.

The first time I recall playing organized sports was when my parents signed me up for T-ball in the summer before kindergarten. At first, I wasn't into it and at times all I would do was swing the bat around like a sword because I wanted to pretend that I was Peter Pan. Other times, I would kick the dirt to make "dirt smoke" or kick the ball like a soccer ball instead of using a bat. Thankfully, I had a coach who was understanding and had a good sense of humour. The thing I liked about T-ball was that I eventually learned to hit a baseball with a bat, something that I had a really difficult time doing since my co-ordination wasn't very good. I didn't know the actual rules of the game for the longest time, and I didn't make long-term friends through this experience, but I did get a small taste of what it was like to be a part of a team.

I played T-ball again in kindergarten, and then I moved on to play soccer for a short time. I think I was inspired to play soccer after seeing it on the TV show *Franklin*. It looked like fun, but I learned it wasn't for me. I wasn't a big fan of playing outside in the heat of summer. I had more fun squirting my teammates with the water bottle than actually playing soccer! This was the first time I wanted to try something new on my own without my parents making me. It was a good thing I gave it a try otherwise I wouldn't have known whether I liked it. Now in my adulthood, I can be reluctant to try new things, but once I push myself outside my comfort zone, I often like them.

As I got older, I moved on to slo-pitch baseball, and I played every spring throughout my school years. I had some great coaches that weren't too competitive, and all my teammates treated me well.

I took swimming and skating lessons as well. Learning how to swim was beneficial, but I didn't like the skating lessons. I already knew how to skate when my parents signed me up. The instructors were disorganized, and I never knew what group I was supposed to be in at the lessons. This was frustrating because I often had the impression that I would get in trouble if I was in the wrong group. I know now that little things like that do not justify punishment, but at the time I didn't.

I was a relatively good swimmer, and I had some decent instructors, but I took a break from lessons occasionally. I was at the indoor pool once when the fire alarm went off. This alarm was much louder than the one at school, and I did not want to go back inside afterward because of my fear of the loud sound. The other time I took a break was after I got a nosebleed during one of the lessons. I didn't want to go back because I thought that my nosebleed was caused by being in the water.

Dad eventually convinced me to go back, and I earned my Bronze Cross in lifeguard training.

My dad and I signed up for karate when I was in Grade 2, and it was the first time we did an organized sport together. Karate was difficult at first, but it helped me control my anger and some of my body movements like hand flapping. The instructors made us stay still for forty-five seconds in the middle of each class. If we moved, we all had to do push-ups. This really helped because it wasn't too harsh of a punishment, and doing the exercises felt good even if I did accidentally move when I wasn't supposed to. It helped me to control my anger because I was able to punch and kick without hitting anyone.

At the end of my first year, I won the "Most Improved Student" award and my first trophy. I wasn't expecting to win anything so it was a big surprise. I was very proud and it made me believe I could accomplish anything. I continued to do karate off and on, eventually earning a yellow belt. Even now I think about taking it up again so I can achieve a black belt someday. Eventually I stopped doing karate because the novelty wore off and I wanted to try other things.

Most Canadian kids want to try hockey, and I was no exception. My dad started a pond hockey league at our local recreation centre so I could play hockey without any pressure. I had mixed feelings about this program. I was upset that it was "play for fun" and not competitive, which was something I wanted. There were times when my parents had to drag me to pond hockey. I guess it's a good thing I never played at the competitive level, as I would never have been able to handle the pressure.

In Grade 4, I developed an interest in basketball. I enjoyed it because I was so tall and blocking shots and shooting seemed to come naturally to me. In Grade 5, I started playing youth basketball in the community. Like most sports I played in my youth, it wasn't overly competitive and was run by coaches who were very encouraging.

My parents were avid squash players, and they asked one of my respite workers and family friend, Sue Nielsen, to include me in her youth squash class, much to my dismay. Sue said I became uncomfortable around large groups of people and excessive noise:

I recall one time Blake left the court holding his ears. I did not realize how loud the vibrational sound from the squash courts were to his ears. I am sorry I put him through that scenario. But I did respect the fact Blake preferred to sit and watch at times.

One time, a kid said something to Blake, and he answered in a forthright manner. That child had such a look of amazement on his face that Blake stood up to his bullying and that he demolished him with his answer. I was proud of Blake.

One undeniable difference between Blake and his peers was his empathy. When other children bullied, Blake spoke kindly. I loved that about him. He never retaliated to the unkind comments that came his way. With his strength and size, he easily could have.

In Grade 7, I wanted to stop playing sports altogether and focus on other things such as video games and theatre. However, my parents pushed me to try out for the basketball team in Grade 8. I did not want to, but they wanted me to experience playing a competitive sport. They said if I didn't like it, I would never have to try out for another school team again. Being given the choice felt good, but I still didn't want to try out. They encouraged me by saying that my cousins enjoyed sports, but this didn't work; in fact, it made me feel like they wanted to change me into someone I wasn't. When I first tried out, I wanted to mess up and pretend I wasn't good at basketball so I wouldn't make the team, but I was afraid of what my parents would do if they found out.

It was a real mystery to me that other kids on the spectrum didn't have parents as pushy as mine. I wondered why my parents couldn't back off and let me do what I felt comfortable doing. As soon as the season started, I could not wait for it to finish. I had a coach that didn't know anything about me and didn't understand what stimming is, let alone when I exhibited it. I also had trouble fitting in with the rest of my teammates. I was so happy when the season ended and relieved that I didn't have to try out for any more sports. In an odd way, I was happy for all the wrong reasons, but I was also proud of myself for going outside my comfort zone and trying something different once again.

Mean Mom, but She Meant Well

Here was my mom's version of the Grade 8 basketball experience from Hell:

> So, he was pretty much the tallest kid in the school. He grew up with a net in his driveway and athletic parents who both played competitive sports. He'd been playing basketball in a fun league where the focus was skill development for four years. They didn't keep score and everyone got equal court time and positive reinforcement. He was HUGE so co-ordination was a work in progress. Stand him under the net and he was guaranteed to make a basket.
>
> When he entered Grade 8, the school board was talking about being inclusive. I pitched to the principal (who, on paper, was supposed to be the boys basketball coach that year) to give Blake a try-out. Much to Blake's reluctance, I pushed for "walk the talk"—I provided articles about other schools that included kids with learning disabilities (LD) on their intercollegiate teams.
>
> Well, for the most part, it was a NIGHTMARE experience I put my son through. In hindsight, I feel awful I forced him to join, but a bit of me is glad I did. Why? Two reasons. First, the team and some of the boys' parents were witness to their sons' bullying exclusion first hand and felt it (albeit from a distance). Second, it added another layer of strength and character to Blake's development. As Grandpa Bud always said, "What doesn't kill you makes you stronger."

Nightmare explained:

The assistant coach was a sixteen-year-old who didn't get why Blake was on the team and had little patience or skill to explain plays to a LD player. He also didn't stop the other players from verbally assaulting Blake when he would act out (mostly due to not understanding). I know it "takes two to tango," but in retrospect it was a set-up for failure for everyone. In the end, it was Blake who suffered most.

The end of season tournament was out of town on a stormy winter weekend. Carpools were arranged, but no one asked or bothered to see if Blake had a ride. First insult, no one noticed that Blake was excluded when they were deciding which boys went in which cars. First game, Blake rode the bench except for a token shift near the end. I get it. I was captain of myriad teams. So does Blake. In between games, the boys all sat together in the hall kibbitzing. Parents milled about a few metres away sipping takeout coffee. Blake tried to physically slide in near the edge. The boys subtly turned their backs. Second insult.

Next game, more of the same.

On the drive home, everyone piled into cars full of three or four boys each. Blake and I drove by ourselves. Thirty minutes into the drive he started to hyperventilate. I stopped the car and he dry-heaved in between sobs. I asked why, but I knew. It turns out that while the team was getting ready for the second game in the change room, a few of the boys had a bit of fun with water bottles. Blake joined in and was quickly shut down.

"You freak."

Third insult.

The final game was the next morning, and the two of us carpooled in silence.

A parent came up to me halfway through the game, tears in her eyes. She told me the boys in her car last night were cutting up Blake behind his back. She was initially oblivious to the verbal bullying and exclusion. (No physical bullying because remember he's HUGE.) She said she was appalled. She stopped her car and reamed them out and said she was ashamed of them all. I thanked her for telling me. I then relayed Blake's version of yesterday's bullying so she could sense his pain.

Blake scored a basket in the final game, and the team all cheered for him. Way to go Blake.

Maybe, after all, each of us learned something from this experience.

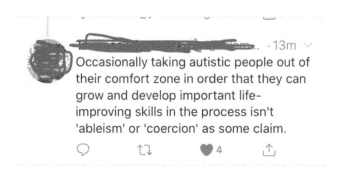

· 13m ⌄

Occasionally taking autistic people out of their comfort zone in order that they can grow and develop important life-improving skills in the process isn't 'ableism' or 'coercion' as some claim.

💬   🔁   ♥ 4   ↑

Tweet emphasizing what my parents believed

I held a grudge against my parents for many years because I didn't know why they made me do something I hated. It's clear now that if they hadn't pushed me outside my comfort zone, I would never have had any new experiences. I would have been in my basement all the time missing out on trying new things. It was something that ultimately prepared me for the life challenges that lay ahead.

In high school, I didn't play any school sports at all. I bowled outside school for a short time, and I really enjoyed it mostly because socializing was easier and it was a lot of fun. Even though I still prefer to watch sports than play them, I am glad I was encouraged to try all these great activities.

The "A" Word—It's Not What You Think!

"The only true award you can receive is being known for doing something that you know is right."

Me

☆

~~Autism~~

~~Accommodations~~

Advocacy

People with autism, whether severe or high functioning[7], are mistreated in schools, public places and by society in general too often. For example, schools make some accommodations for students who are severely autistic, but they often don't provide accommodations to those who appear less challenged. Do they think that high-functioning autism is "easy" autism? This couldn't be further from the truth. In fact, without supports and accommodations, autism isn't easy at all.

I was lucky that the schools I went to came to their senses and provided me with the accommodations I needed to be successful. However, I was only offered them after my mom and dad were rather persistent at stating the obvious: that their kid needed support to meet his educational goals. They were like a dog with a bone, and when being nice didn't work, they threatened the school board with legal action for not respecting my rights. I am sure my parents could write

---

[7]   "High-functioning" is a term I talk more about in Chapter 5.

an entire book on all the stuff they have done over the years. It is really unfair that any parents need to go through so much crap just so their kid receives a decent education.

Elementary School Advocacy

I was too young to understand all the "behind the scenes" things my parents did at my elementary school to help me succeed. I sat in on a lot of meetings. My special ed teacher, Robin Spry, recalled:

> Blake's parents fought tirelessly on his behalf. They saw his potential and would stop at nothing to ensure he received all the support and help he deserved. And they did it with integrity and kindness, wisdom and professionalism. Fortunately, all their hard work EVENTUALLY paid off. Never before, nor since, have I seen the school board step up and provide what a student needed like they did for Blake. Sad. The threat of a lawsuit can do wonders! LOL!

My mom was at the school a lot and not just as a parent volunteer. Here's a bit about her experience advocating for me in elementary school:

> Well, I was like a momma bear protecting her cub. We were fortunate that we had the resources to put into the fight. It did come with sacrifices. When Blake was in senior kindergarten, I quit my job when Ted and I realized that in order for him to have a positive school experience, he would need a visible, active advocate in the school's face. Thankfully, I had a very understanding boss (Louise!) who refused to accept my resignation and offered part-time flexible work instead. So, for five years we took a major hit with reduced family income, pension and benefits, but it was a small price to pay to ensure Blake was safe and learning at school.

In order to figure out this new educational system, Ted and I needed to infiltrate the system to determine Blake's legal rights. Ted joined the school Parent Involvement Committee for a few years, actively chaired the anti-bullying group and played "good cop" at Identification, Placement and Review Committee (IPRC) meetings while I played "bad cop" with tears and much foul language. I spent time on the school board's Special Education Advisory Committee (SEAC) representing rural parents of kids with autism. We met wonderful, committed educators, trustees, parents, self-advocates and bureaucrats on these committees. What often came out of our experience at these tables was, "We agree he needs X, but we don't have the resources/allocation…" blah, blah, blah. Not the right answer!

So, for several years while Blake was in elementary school, Ted and I would request and/or facilitate meetings at the school with invited decision makers like the director of education, various superintendents, our local trustee, principal, vice-principal, special education teacher, classroom teacher, local health and social services provider and sometimes other parents of kids with ASD. We wanted Blake to be present at most of these meetings so they could see we were talking about a real little person. We'd send out agendas and briefing notes in advance and expect solution-oriented answers. Most times we were dreaming in technicolour, but sometimes we'd win a fight.

Imagine fighting for what is simply a right? If Blake had been blind or in a wheelchair the accommodations would have been more easily put in place. Having an invisible disability put Blake and his friend Jakob at a distinct disadvantage. Without sustained parental pressure there probably would have been no accommodations and supports.

Rural schools in an urban school board end up with crumbs for resources. Blake's school administration and staff realized early on that we were their allies and were advocating on their behalf, not against them. This change of perspective only came about with considerable, consistent efforts at developing trusting relationships with all parties. This took an inordinate amount of time given the constant turnover at the school and board levels.

When Blake was in Grade 3, I co-presented with the director of education about the "Inequity of Education" at a Human Rights Commission Hearing in North Bay. I used Blake's school situation as the example. I always thought I could use my voice to change the system so it would be better for all those who didn't have a voice or the resources to fight for their educational rights.

We met MPs and MPPs when Blake was young— Senator Jim Munson, Brent St. Denis and, more recently, Mike Mantha and Carol Hughes. They all know Blake's story and the inequities facing those who live in rural northern communities.

There were times when I had to focus my anger (a.k.a. advocacy efforts) at making sure Blake got what he needed and to hell with anyone else. I know it sounds selfish, but he often fell through the cracks because he was a well-behaved, quiet kid. We fought unsuccessfully for four years (grades 1-4) to get him support from an EA to work on social communication goals during structured and unstructured times.

We privately hired Jakob's mom, Vicky, to support Blake at lunchtime at school. Initially, the principal would not allow Vicky on the schoolyard. We argued that it was in his IPRC and IEP to have this support, so either provide it or fuck off we will. Oh, by the way, please ensure the school's insurance policy covers Vicky. So Vicky supervised Blake for a few years during lunchtime in the yard. This gave Ted and me peace of mind that Blake was safe, and it gave Vicky a chance to watch her son (Jakob) from a distance too. Autism parents stick together!

Our house had a big filing cabinet full of my documentation. My mom kept all my school IEPs, IPRCs, psychological, occupational, physical, speech and language assessments, applications for respite grants, disability credits and supports. She seemed to always be filling out forms on my behalf.

Sue Nielsen, our family friend, shared more of her reflections on the advocacy challenges my parents endured:

> I will never forget when the heartache and challenges of autism fully struck home for me. I recall it so well. Jo and I were good friends, and we chatted often and went on walks, etc. We compared notes about the school Blake and my daughter attended. We talked about the challenges they were facing in securing special education support for Blake. At that point he was in a regular classroom at the back of the room and not getting the help he needed.
>
> Because of budgetary cutbacks or philosophical differences between Blake's parents and the school board, Blake was being left out. Jo started to cry—it was the first time I had ever seen her cry. She was extremely frustrated with the process of having to go above and beyond at the school and with the board. But I sensed

her overall frustration in dealing with people who did not understand the world of an autistic child and the challenges it presented.

It all came out that day, and it was actually quite beautiful because I saw her humanity and her love for her child, and the disgust she felt at how a system can discriminate against children with special needs. I had been oblivious to Blake's parents' pain and frustration, so this conversation was an epiphany and a valuable insight I never forgot. I understood the heartache, frustration, weariness and anger Jo and Ted felt. They did everything in their power to ensure he had equal treatment at school and in the community, and they paid an emotional price for that.

I don't recall there being any support systems for parents of autistic children at that time in our community. Raising a child with autism in our small town was a constant challenge; it was exhausting, exhilarating and lonely for parents. Blake is blessed to have parents who support him, and they are blessed to have a child like him. I was blessed to know Blake and to have loved him as his caregiver and friend.

High School Advocacy

My mom's advocacy efforts for my Grade 9 placement began when I was in Grade 7. I guess she knew that these things take time. Without accommodations, things would have been much more difficult, and it could have meant that I went to high school for six years instead of four. It was thanks to my mom that I was able to attend Espanola High School (EHS) in my hometown with teachers who knew about autism and could spend time with me to ensure I got my work done and could be successful. The school board wanted to send all EHS's autistic kids to a Sudbury high school because they had dumped most of the special education resources there. My mom said that this would be grounds for discrimination. It would also have been really difficult for me to travel over seventy kilometres to school. I wouldn't have had the energy to work a part-time job or participate in any extracurricular activities.

The school system often used "lack of money" as an excuse for not providing me with the services I needed, but they were less likely to refuse accommodations for someone with a visible physical disability. It's really sad that people on the spectrum or people with invisible disabilities aren't treated fairly.

In Grade 8, I didn't understand why my mom was having me tour other high schools in Sudbury, an hour's drive away. I thought for the longest time she was being an overprotective mother, and I didn't understand until I got older that she was obtaining information to prove that there was sufficient need for a comprehensive ASD resource program for all autistic students at EHS. So that is another school board battle she led. She helped convince the board to provide the necessary supports at our local high school instead of bussing us down the TransCanada Highway every day outside of our hometown. I owe a lot to my mom.

While these advocacy battles my parents fought got me the educational support, they also advocated on behalf of other autistic families. They focused on levelling the playing field in various systems— mainly lack of access in northern rural communities in education, and health and social services. My mom got pretty good at making protest signs and meeting politicians, but she was constantly frustrated with the lack of action that resulted.

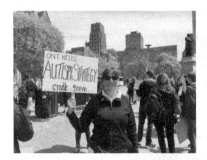
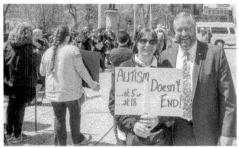
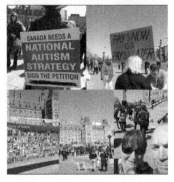

Provincial and federal peaceful protests my parents participated in about lack of strategies and funding for autism community

My elementary years were a huge challenge. I learned how to communicate socially, get along with classmates and participate in community activities all while pushing myself out of my comfort zone.

My teen years took me through a whole new level of challenges. Read on to hear how I didn't just survive but thrived in high school!

Chapter 3:

My Teen Years: Surviving and Thriving in High School

Time to Become a Spartan

High school is the best years of some kids' lives while others just want to forget it. The Barenaked Ladies song "Grade 9" details those struggles, but nothing they sing about happened to me. No, high school for me was not about wet willies and swirlies; it was struggling with difficult subjects, relationships and bullies.

The first week at EHS, home of the Spartans, went pretty well. I met my teachers and gained an understanding of what to expect in the courses. I spent an hour or so each day in the ASD resource room where I could do my work, take a sensory break or talk about problems. Having the ASD classroom led by Mr. Diebel, a.k.a. Mr. D, was so beneficial. I had people who knew me and understood that I learn differently.

One of the first things I had to learn was to talk like other teens. I recall telling a bully in my class that he was "going the right way for a smacked bottom" (a line from the movie *Shrek*). My EA heard and told me that it was not something that teenagers say to one another, and she took the time to teach me what I should say. I didn't know how to talk in a way that other teenagers did because I had spent a lot more time with adults than I had with kids my own age up until that point. I felt more comfortable around adults because they were more mature and I could relate to them better. Kids my age were noisy and immature.

Bullying wasn't a huge problem for me in high school probably because I was huge, though there were some occasional incidents. One time I was walking down the hall to my class and some idiot decided it would be funny to trip me. It wasn't funny at all, but I didn't get too mad. I just gave him a dirty look and walked away. I was concerned that it would happen again, only next time it would be worse. My teachers and EAs assured me there were cameras around the school, so if I was ever bullied they would be able to find out who did it. They said I shouldn't be afraid to tell someone. I was still worried that if I told I would be called a snitch and the bullying would intensify. Later, my parents told me that if bullies got upset that I told on them it's their problem because they brought it on themselves.

My parents recall that bullying was less prominent in high school than in elementary school as well. But it wasn't totally absent from my life. Subtle exclusion and shunning still happened, but I was learning to not take it to heart. It was also difficult to be accepted into a group or social situations in Grade 9. One time at Spartan Youth Radio (SYR), the only extracurricular program I was involved with, a student bought a pizza for everyone but me. I was never offered a piece, which made me feel left out. I had no idea why I wasn't included.

Misreading an unwritten social rule, misinterpreting conversations, or unintentionally staring too long at someone can escalate into trouble. Often it is a simple misunderstanding. Mr. D recalled several times that made him sad.

> When Blake went out to different classes sometimes the rate of social interactions and the topics confused and upset him. In helping him understand what was said or demonstrated, I often felt sad that it affected Blake in this way as he was really struggling with what took place. Fortunately, these occurrences got less and less frequent as Blake adapted to the different environments and applied coping skills.

My mom drove me to and from school for years because the school bus is a great place for bullies to ply their trade. I know I'm not alone in this belief. My two lifelong neighbour friends, the Brown's, took the same bus so I had allies to watch out for me, but sometimes they weren't on the bus so I had to fend for myself. I tried lots of strategies—from sitting at the front to wearing headphones to tune out the taunting. My enormous size in high school eventually shut down the bullying for the most part. By the time I started Grade 10, most of my peers had matured enough to start accepting me into school project groups, which made me feel much better.

Fitting in wasn't my only challenge in high school. I also struggled with certain subjects. I had a really difficult time understanding complicated math—the kind of math no one needs to know in their everyday life. Geometry and trigonometry stumped me. At times, the struggle was so stressful that I was worried I wouldn't pass. Math had never been my best subject in school, and I needed to get my three required credits over with as soon as possible. I started by taking a math course in the first semester of Grade 9, and it wasn't so hard. But the following semester I took a nightmare Grade 10 math course. No matter what I did I could not understand the material, and I always needed help. It was so bad that at times I was very stressed out and worried that I would have to take the course again. I wasn't being challenged academically—it was my sanity that was being tested instead! In the end, I passed the course with a 70%.

After that, I decided that my last math course would be beneficial for my everyday life. So Mr. Diebel and I agreed that I should take the Workplace and Everyday Life math course where I would learn about paying bills, taxes and banking. However, my mentor and tutor, Sandy Hayden, felt it would be too easy for me and she tried to push me to take a college prep course instead. I know now that she meant well because she believed I could do anything. I had to be firm and tell her I knew what I wanted to do in my future and I didn't need to learn more trigonometry, calculus or geometry to get there. I think she was disappointed at first but she later accepted my decision. The workplace math wasn't as easy as Sandy had predicted, and I still needed help now and then, but I finished the course with a 69%, a bit lower than my Grade 10 mark.

Sandy remembered all the math struggles we both went through as she tutored me:

> Blake believed he could not do math, but I knew he could. We managed to get to grade level by the end of Grade 8. In high school Blake was really struggling with math, and I could not understand why he couldn't grasp the material he had successfully worked through in Grade 8. One day it dawned on me. I told him he needed to bring all of the lessons he learned in elementary school with him to high school so he could build on them. I explained that it was about "boxes." The stuff inside the first box was necessary for the

second box—you could not do it without it. This
analogy clicked! All of a sudden, he was doing very
well in math! However, he still did not like it and still
believed he was not very good at it (not true at all).

Blake has a wonderful mind, and watching it work is
absolutely amazing.

Math wasn't the only course I struggled with in high school. Grades
9 and 10 English were difficult as well. English was typically one of my
best subjects, but I had the same teacher two years in a row. He was nice,
but he was extremely difficult to impress because his expectations were
too high for an applied English course. One time I made a movie poster
that he was not impressed with so he gave me a low mark. I felt that it
was the best I could do, so I wanted to settle for the low mark, but the
EA convinced me that I could do better. She said she would help me
make a better poster that would earn me a better mark. I was reluctant
to do this, but my English mark was already low and my dad had told
me I needed high English marks to get into media and journalism. So,
I decided to try making the poster again.

In the end, I earned a better mark and that teacher's expectations
inspired me to try even harder in the future. I learned I should never
accept a mark, even if it is a passing grade, if I can do better. During
the rest of my high school career, I chose to work as hard as I possibly
could and it certainly paid off! I made it on the honour roll four times,
and when I graduated, I went home with three bursaries. I would never
have achieved this without the encouragement I needed to be my best.

One of my favourite teachers of all time, Mr. D, reflected on my
time at EHS.

What was different about Blake? I guess the best word
to describe him was "guarded," not fearful. I had not
earned his trust or respect at that point so he needed to
sum me up. Blake was physically taller than most, and
his body language reflected his emotions. He surprised
me how quickly he engaged with his peers. With so

many new experiences in the first month, he had some challenges, but he quickly learned he could talk to an EA or me. He was encouraged to take the time needed to process the challenges, and with guidance from us, he developed many coping mechanisms. In comparison to his ASD classmates, he was the most socially engaging. The class environment with peers with similar challenges seemed to allow him to be himself. Blake was keen to go to his different classes and quickly realized he had a safe place to come back to if needed.

As far as traits, I would say Blake was a processor. When challenges or change (positive or negative) arose he needed to think, ask questions and process the information. As mentioned earlier, his body language spoke volumes. Awareness was a great coping strategy for him.

When Blake came to EHS, one of his biggest concerns was the dreaded fire alarm. This sprouted from the unnecessary sound used in elementary school to distinguish the message from school bells. When he was assured that in the high school the alarm was a simple three chirp bell sound, he was still very anxious. We made sure he was in the ASD room for the first drill, and when it sounded, he looked up and I said we had to exit the building as part of the drill. Blake was amazed by how "wimpy" the bell was.

"That's it? That's all there is?" he asked.

Blake never feared a fire drill again!

When Blake was focused on a task, he blocked out peers. But he showed them he cared when he saw them in distress, quickly acknowledging them and, of course, offering them advice on how to deal with the problem. Blake was equally quick to defend a peer if a fellow classmate was dishing out unjust criticism. As well, if a peer was being a distraction to him and bothering others as well, Blake had no problem joining in and letting the student know how he felt.

We laughed almost every day as Blake has a good sense of humour and could recite many quotes from different movies and television shows. I also like to look at life from the lighter side, so we had lots of fun jeering with each other.

The best tools to help Blake were awareness, time and talking it out in the counselling room free from distractions and away from his peers.

I am proud of what Blake has accomplished. There will always be change and challenges, but I am sure he will overcome them. Our four years together at EHS are ones I reflect on warmly.

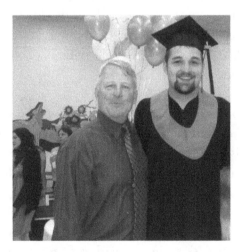

Mr. D and me at graduation—both very happy!

The best part of working with Mr. D was that he taught me to have a positive outlook on life. A few of the teachers I had didn't seem very fond of their jobs, and if they won the lottery, they would quit teaching. Not Mr. D. He was the stark opposite. He really enjoyed his job and because of that he helped to make my time at high school better and easier. He even made me a fan of Mondays to a degree! He had a great sense of humour that really helped get us through the day. He liked telling goofy and sometimes off-colour jokes and would answer the classroom phone in a funny way.

"City morgue. You stab 'em we slab 'em."

Best of all, he helped all of us when we were overwhelmed or distressed. I am very blessed to have had the chance to know him.

Becoming a Teen Ain't Easy—for Everyone

My mom said when *typical* kids are about thirteen years old, they become self-absorbed and break away from their parents to find their place in the peer group. I went through this phase, but later than my peers. My mom shared what this stage was like:

> What we witnessed was withdrawal of support and engagement from his peers. Peer Buddies engaged and played the previous few years, but this decreased by Grade 7. It wasn't a problem with Blake, but mere typical teen development.

> The phone no longer rang for get-togethers. It was difficult to hear what Blake's peer group was doing— going fishing, playing pick-up basketball, paintball, house parties. I'm not sure if Blake felt the exclusion. It was subtle, but it sure pained me.

> On Blake's thirteenth birthday, he was at school eating lunch at his desk trying so hard to fit in and be social. He said to a female classmate, "You look good enough to eat." Instant gasps and laughter at Blake's faux pas.

From what the teacher pieced together, this was a saying the EA regularly said to her three-year-old daughter in an innocent display of affection. Blake, not reading the context, ended up saying what turned into a sexual connotation comment to a female classmate. I picked him up at school shortly after the incident. He was in tears—embarrassed, confused and exhausted from the rejection. With tears in my eyes, I said to the teacher, "Can't he just have one normal day of being treated nicely?" I no longer used the word "normal," but the teacher knew what I meant. Just a day without unwritten social rules exploding in his face.

Speaking of unwritten social rules, many of Blake's IEP goals throughout his fourteen years of school were focused on social skills. We figured he could always use a calculator to handle math deficits, but if he didn't learn how to converse and actively listen, he'd be hard pressed to be successfully independent. We live in a social world, and while there's merit in individuality and quirkiness, sometimes in order to attain one's life goals "we gotta fake it till we make it." Current literature and first hand accounts of how exhausting it is to mask and camouflage and learn all these social skills and rules have me realizing today that all this comes with an emotional price. I'm still grappling with this conundrum. Blake talks more about this in Chapter 5.

Unwritten Social Rules and What Happens if Not Followed

So, I've been taught the following social rules:
- Don't invade people's space. That means don't get too close to them;
- Don't stare at someone (no matter how good looking they are!);
- Don't make comments about anyone's bodies, good or bad;

- Don't tell dirty, sexual or racist jokes;
- Don't hug or touch anyone unless they are part of your family or they have agreed to be your boy/girlfriend and you have both agreed to it.

Then I watch real life unfold, and I am confused.

When I'm with my cousins and friends, we tell dirty jokes and make the occasional inappropriate comment. Teens and adults will often touch someone when they are not a family member. It seems that there are exceptions to these rules which are unwritten and not easy to decode.

It would help if every community was autism-friendly and inclusive. Channel-Port aux Basques, Newfoundland, a place I would love to live, is the first autism-friendly town in Canada. One focus is on autism sensitivity training for first responders (police officers, ambulance attendants, bus drivers, lifeguards) to ensure safety of their autistic citizens. My mom and dad attended similar training years ago by Dennis Debbaudt, a Florida father who started a training program because his autistic teen son had been approached by a police officer while out for a walk by himself on a sunny day in his neighbourhood. It was an unexpected encounter, and his son didn't react "normally." He didn't make eye contact so he must be guilty, right? He ended up in the back of the cruiser. It could have gotten worse, but it was enough of a red flag for Dennis to realize he needed to do something so it wouldn't happen again to his son and all the other innocent autistic folks out there.

How do we learn all these unwritten social rules? Autistics often learn the hard way. The onus needs to be on everyone to learn. The Social Model of Disability in Chapter 5 states the environment needs to be changed, not the autistic person. All communities should provide autism sensitivity training, starting with first responders.

Working Past the False Shame of Autism

In the previous chapter I talked about the severe anxiety I had to deal with in elementary school, but my teen years brought on a new set of problems. Because I was going through puberty, little things that happened felt like the end of the world. The anxiety was bad, but it wasn't as bad as the depression I felt. When I worried, it was about things that teenagers commonly worry about: grades, whether a girl you like is attracted to you—that sort of thing. My depression, on the other hand, was unbearable at times. I felt ashamed of who I was for having autism because I was different from other students, and I often blamed my autism for my lack of a girlfriend.

I had been on a few "dates," like at the elementary school graduation dance and the Halloween dance, but I had never had any serious relationships. I was under the impression that no girls would ever want to go out with me if they knew I was on the spectrum, so this made me wish I wasn't in the ASD class so I could keep my autism a secret. There was this one girl I desperately tried to impress, but she was dating another kid. I went too far trying to get her to notice me, and she told my teacher, so I was told to stop bothering her. I decided I would respect her feelings. She said we were already friends and she wanted us to be like brother and sister. I felt better knowing that the reason she didn't want to go out with me had nothing to do with my autism.

Sadly, this wasn't the end of my teenage depression. I knew there were other fish in the sea, but I didn't think I would be happy until I had a girlfriend and lost my virginity. I thought everyone else at school was getting intimate, so I should be too.

Sometimes the stress of being a teenager was too much to bear, and I felt as though my life wasn't worth living. When you're a teenager and you have all these hormones to deal with, it all just seems like the end of the world. As an adult, things like this don't bother me as much, but when you're young you often focus on what's happening now rather than looking forward to the future. I told my parents and teachers that I was unhappy with my life and that I wanted to commit suicide, something I had never thought of doing before. I wanted my life to end because I was autistic and single, and I was sure I wasn't going to amount to anything. I figured I wouldn't be missed because I was already a burden to my family. My parents had to convince me that killing myself would be a mistake because not only would I not have a second chance at life, but I would also hurt everyone else that cared about and loved me. I didn't believe what they said because I was focused on my own pain; I hadn't considered how my friends and family would feel. It wasn't until a student at my high school committed suicide that I realized just how wrong I was to even consider taking my own life. I attended the girl's funeral and saw just how devastated her friends and family were. I understood then that taking your own life doesn't take the pain away, it passes it on to everyone else.

Grandma Dot used to say, "This too shall pass," which means things will get better in the future. And they sure have.

Some of you reading this book may be severely depressed and feeling as though life isn't worth living. If you are contemplating suicide, remember this: feeling pain is a good thing. It means you're still alive and being alive is the best feeling of all. If you're alive and breathing, your life is far from ruined. If you feel that no one loves you or cares about you, they do. Even in darkness, all human beings are loved. Never, ever be afraid to ask for help. Never be afraid to show your emotions. It takes a lot more courage and bravery to ask for help and let your emotions out than it does to keep it all a secret.

Travelling and Seeing New Places

Ecuador: The first time I left North America was in 2008 when we took a family trip to Ecuador. We prepared for this trip by taking Spanish lessons and watching documentaries about the Amazon and the Galapagos Islands so we knew what to expect. I took to it right away because I was eager to visit another continent.

This trip marked the first time I'd experience a whole new culture, and I spent a lot of time preparing by learning about unwritten social rules. I learned that some of the social rules in Ecuador were completely different than those I was used to in Canada. Learning these new social rules helped me understand the customs of different people and develop a sense of tolerance.

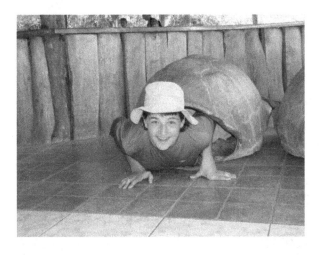

Not every day you can hide in a tortoise shell, Galapagos, Ecuador, 2008

The Galapagos Islands were the highlight of the trip for all of us. Being on a small boat in the Pacific Ocean for a week with twenty people was amazing! We went snorkelling with seals, penguins and sharks, ate delicious food and spent hours gazing up at the vast night-time stars. I only had one blip on the whole trip. It's funny that none of us remember what the trigger was. Here's what Kristen, my family friend, recalled:

> One day during our trip to the Galapagos, Blake was upset on the boat. What he did then and still does now (and I think it works well for him!) was pace the deck and process his thoughts. He would walk in circles trying to understand his anger and the situation. Eventually he came around and his spirits perked up!

After Galapagos, we flew into the heart of the Amazon. Being Canadians and used to the cold, a hot and humid jungle was completely new. This adventure helped me prepare for the times in life that are unpredictable and are a real test of my sanity. Sometimes I hear about parents who give their kids a loving push outside their comfort zone to help prepare them for the unexpected in life, but in this case we all went outside our comfort zones. I went more outside my comfort zone than most kids on the spectrum in this situation!

So why are jungles so intense, and why was this particular adventure hard?

We quickly learned just how alive the jungle was with creatures, bugs and spiders as big as your hand! The scenery was intensely beautiful. Our hike was by far the most intense one I have ever been on. Not only were there creepy, deadly insects and wildlife but the humidity was unbearable. I already have a severe heat sensitivity, but this was like being in a sauna turned on full on the hottest day of the year while wearing a parka and a toque (winter hat)! It was all worth it though because we got to see some cool creatures like monkeys, exotic birds, a tortoise and tracks of ocelots, tapirs and armadillos.

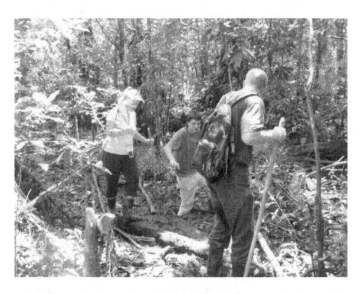

**Stuck in mud halfway through a five-hour
Amazon jungle hike with 100% humidity**

Vancouver: The next big trip for the three of us was going to Vancouver for the Winter Olympics in 2010. While at the Olympics, I got a chance to practise my on-air skills. I was involved with Spartan Youth Radio, a media club at my high school, and I called them live from the events so they could follow what was going on. That was a cool opportunity.

Nova Scotia: Next, we did a road trip to the east coast of Canada, starting with a few days in Ottawa for Canada Day celebrations. I had been to Ottawa a few times before, but this was the first time we spent Canada Day in our nation's capital. It was a hot day and we were surrounded by over a million people on Parliament Hill, but I managed to do fine because it was something I wanted to do.

Before leaving Ottawa and heading east, we were invited to a friend's house for supper where I made two social mistakes. The first one happened when they served vegetarian lasagna, something I am not able to stomach. My parents had prepared me in advance that I might be served food I can't tolerate. I was supposed to just play with it on my plate, and they would go through a drive through on the way back to the hotel! I managed to pretend to eat it, and I even told them that it was good, but when they asked if I wanted more, I told them a bit too loudly and firmly 'NO!' Whoops.

The other social mistake I made was telling them their living room looked like the *Titanic*. My parents explained that someone could misunderstand and assume I was saying it was ugly, like the wreck of the *Titanic*. After that, I learned to be more careful when making comments. We laugh about this now.

We stayed in a refurbished train car in Tatamagouche, Nova Scotia. I have always been a fan of trains, so I enjoyed this. We met up with Lanny, Eliza and Grace and did all sorts of fun things together like whale watching, hiking and swimming. In Halifax, we saw the boats in the harbour, but one of my favourites was *Theodore Too*, a replica of Theodore Tugboat from the 1990s TV series. I felt like going for a ride on *Theodore Too*, but at the same time I was worried that I would be made fun of for going on a ride meant for kids, so I just got my photo taken with Theodore instead. If I had the chance to go for a ride on *Theodore Too* now, I would certainly go because I know now that I shouldn't worry about what other people think. If I enjoy something I should just go ahead and do it. As long as it's legal.

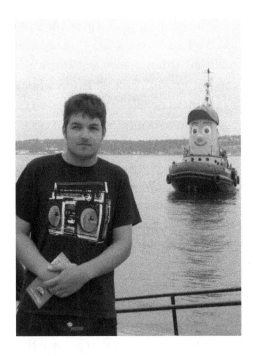

**Never too old for a childhood blast from
the past! Halifax, Nova Scotia**

At one point my parents and I decided to split up and do our own
thing, so I took a bus to a mall. When it was time to go back to the
hotel, I ended up taking the wrong bus which went to the suburbs far
away from downtown Halifax. I was really embarrassed. I was also
afraid about what would happen once the bus driver made me get off,
but he said that he would pick me up after his break. I was so anxious
about being lost that I got upset with him out of fear and frustration.
I decided to walk to a nearby corner store thinking I would call a
cab instead of taking the bus. That's when I ran into the bus driver.
Without thinking, I got upset and angry with him again, and because
of my behaviour he refused to give me a ride back. I was thankful to
the workers at the store because they agreed to call me a cab. I told
them I thought people on the east coast were supposed to be friendly
and if I had ever treated a customer the way the bus driver had treated
me, I would have gotten in trouble. I had been taught at my grocery
store job that the customer is always right. I would later learn that if a

customer is making a worker feel uncomfortable, they have the right to walk away. I had no intention of making anyone feel bad, I just did not know what to say and do because I was scared. This situation caused angst for my parents as well:

> Waiting in our hotel room, the clock ticking—where is Blake? He should have been back hours ago. We were both silently nervous, thinking worst-case scenarios. After what seemed like an eternity, Blake finally called us…we met him stepping out from the front seat of a cab…we paid the fare (huge!) and hugged Blake. That evening over seafood, he unravelled the incident. Another perspective-taking learning experience chocked up! We chatted and role-played about what he would do differently next time.

Even though this part of the trip was uncomfortable and scary, it taught me what I should do and how I should act if that ever happened again. When we got back home, I started to wear my autism/anxiety medical alert bracelet and put its accompanying information card in my wallet. My bracelet reminds me to stay calm, and the card gives tips to others in case they need to help de-escalate a potential situation.

New York City and England: The following summer I went to England with a group of eight American autistic young adults, chaperoned by three psychologists. Since the group would be flying out of New York City, my parents and I decided to go there a few days before my departure. We visited Ground Zero, the Statue of Liberty, Radio City Music Hall, Times Square, Central Park and, of course, Yankee Stadium, where we took in a ball game.

My ability to handle unexpected changes gets stronger every time I'm with my parents! On the way to the ball game my mom got us lost in Harlem and it took two cabs to get us to the Bronx. On the way back she picked the wrong subway line headed for Coney Island instead of our Central Park stop. We laughed, and I said, "Well, I've always wanted to try a Coney dog!"

At the JFK Airport, I met the group I would be travelling with. I didn't really notice any autistic characteristics. My dad remembered a sweet interaction that day. "As the group was mingling with introductions, we parents were on the peripheral. I overheard two of the young adults start a conversation—something to the effect of, "Oh, you will fit right in—you have British teeth."

Before we boarded the plane, I gave everyone a maple sugar candy I had brought from Canada, something I think they all enjoyed. We arrived in London around six in the morning local time. We were all very tired after the journey, and it was difficult to get used to the time difference.

We stayed in an old country-style hotel with a nice garden. After a nap, we went out for supper to an Italian restaurant before taking in *Billy Elliot* the musical. During the meal I started to feel overwhelmed because I was in a different country with a bunch of people I didn't know and I was still suffering from jet leg. I started crying a little bit and was a bit shaky. One of the group leaders helped me by having me take deep breaths and by giving me a back rub. This helped a little bit, but I started to think I had bitten off more than I could chew and this trip was a bad idea. The group leaders told me that after a good night's sleep I would feel better, and they were right. The next morning I felt like a new man, totally refreshed and ready for adventure. I was happy to be on the trip again.

We spent the day touring all the famous sites of London like the Elizabeth Tower, also known as Big Ben, and Buckingham Palace. Our next stop was Oxford, Winston Churchill's birth place, and Stonehenge. To this day I still wonder how the ancient Saxons or Celtics managed to put those stones in place without machinery.

We spent the second last day of the trip in Stratford-upon-Avon, the place to go if you like theatre, especially Shakespearian theatre. The highlight of the trip was seeing *Macbeth* in a traditional Shakespearian-style theatre. It made my theatre mentor back home very jealous.

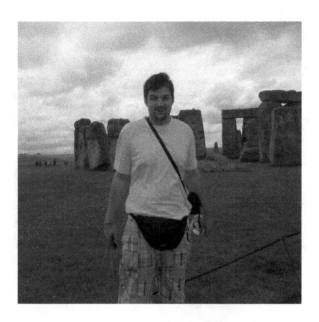

An engineering marvel, Stonehenge, England

Italy: The next year, my high school announced there would be an organized trip to Italy in the spring of 2012. My parents agreed they would pay for half of the trip, and I paid the other half by working my part-time job at the grocery store. Once the trip was paid for in full, the organizer and the school guidance counsellor sat me down and told me what to expect. One important thing she told me was that when we had free time to go exploring, I had to be with another student. I was a bit unsure of that at first, but once I found out that people I knew would be on the trip I felt a little better. The night before the trip I was really nervous and had butterflies in my stomach. I couldn't understand why because I had done this before and I should have been excited, but my parents said it was common to feel nervous.

A lot of the students were nervous, and I tried to help them through it since I knew what it was like to travel overseas. Many of the students had never even been on a plane before.

Our first stop was Verona, the setting for *Romeo and Juliet*. We also visited Venice, a beautiful city on the Mediterranean Sea with amazing architecture. Other places we toured included Pompeii, Florence, Pisa, Rome and Vatican City.

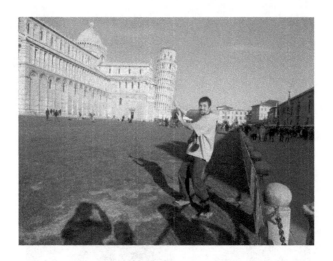

Pushing on the Leaning Tower of Pisa

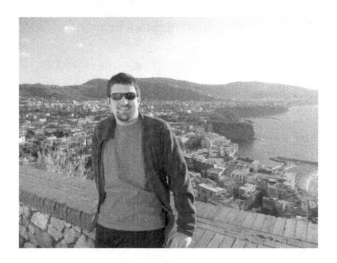

Taking in the Italian scenery

Like all trips, sometimes bad things happen. Toward the end of the trip, I became quite anxious when I heard some of the kids were planning to have a few drinks on the last day. My roommate even offered me a beer. I had drunk alcohol before so that wasn't the problem. I was the only one that was of legal drinking age on the trip but because it was a school trip, we were not allowed to drink alcohol. If we did drink, we could get sent home or get suspended from school.

My mind was racing when I was offered the drink. I wanted to have a beer, but at the same time I didn't want to get in trouble. Before this trip, the school had said they were not going to be organizing a senior prom because some kids had brought alcohol to the Valentine's Day dance, and this did not go over very well with the students. I was concerned that if a bunch of kids got drunk on this trip it could mean that the school would not organize any more trips to Europe. This would not be fair to everyone else, and I wanted other students to experience what I got to see and do.

I decided to walk away and think, but that didn't work. I started breathing heavily and fell to the floor in distress. One of the girls on the trip gave me a back rub and asked me what was wrong, but I didn't feel comfortable telling her (though it did feel good to have her comfort me). We found a teacher I was comfortable talking to (I had known this man since the beginning of high school), and I told him what happened. I also said I was scared that if the other kids found out that I snitched on them I would never be able to show my face in the school again. He told me not to worry and that they would pretend they didn't know about it. He also told me how proud he was of me for being so mature for my age and for knowing that there is a time and a place to do things such as drinking.

Calgary: After graduating from high school, I got to go to the 100th Calgary Stampede and stay with my close family friends, Leigh and John. The stampede is one of those events everyone must go to at least once. We rode the Ferris wheel, took in some calf roping and ate too many deep-fried Oreo cookies. We took a day trip to Banff to hike a mountain that had a beautiful glacial lake at the top. I feel fortunate to have had the opportunity to see this part of Canada.

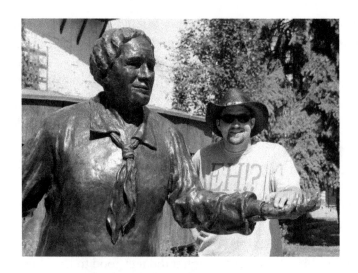

**Hanging out with my Famous Five relative, Emily Murphy,
while in Calgary at the Stampede** *(courtesy L. McAdam)*

Wilderness Survival School: For graduation, my parents gifted
me a week at the Wilderness Survival School. I had been a fan of Les
Stroud, a.k.a. *Survivorman,* for a long time, and I wanted to go because
it was the same program he had taken before becoming famous. In this
course we would have to make fires without matches, sleep in shelters
and find our own food. If you like the outdoors like I do, it's important
to know some basic survival skills. My brother from another mother,
Cam came with me on this trip. This was not the first time Cam and I
had done bush craft and outdoor activities together as he and his dad,
Bim, taught me a lot about fishing and hunting.

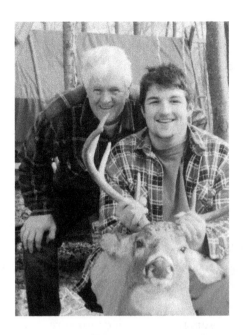

**My main hunting and fishing mentor, Bim with
my first buck "Bimbo"** *(courtesy V. & B. Adams)*

This experience was way better than any summer camp I had ever gone to. On the first day the instructor took us for a walk to show us some edible and poisonous plants. We also spent time getting to know the other participants. One of the instructors at the school was on the autism spectrum as well, and he was a good teacher who knew a lot about the wilderness and survival.

We slept in tents and heard the soothing sounds of nature and wolves howling for the first two nights. One of my first challenges was when we had pasta for supper. I tried eating it without the sauce, and though that helped I still had trouble swallowing it. They say, "Beggars can't be choosers," but it's another story when you can't keep the food down!

When it came time to sleep in a shelter, it felt good to walk in the footsteps of Les Stroud. Even though the first two nights were rainy and foul it was still an exciting experience for me. I think I enjoyed the shelters better than the tent, though it was difficult to sleep on the hard ground without a sleeping bag. It felt good when I contributed to the group by collecting firewood and materials for our shelter, and I even started a fire without matches. I never got a fire going by rubbing two sticks together, but I did get one going with a flint and some hand sanitizer.

After eating bland carbs for days, I was looking forward to eating real food at home. That's when I realized how thankful I was to have my home and family. Many people in Canada and other countries around the world don't. I had something to look forward to when I got home, but many people don't have that option; they have to eat bread and beans and rice every day or sometimes nothing at all. The trip made me realize that I shouldn't take anything for granted in life and that some first world problems really aren't problems at all.

Cam told his version of one of our adventures, which was my favourite part of the week:

> It was a real survival experience for sure, and it poured rain for two days!! It was the middle of the summer, but we still endured sleepless, wet, cold nights. One night we heard howling and realized our site was close to a wolf den! Were we an easy meal?
>
> A day and half went by, and food was tight. We did have rice if needed. Blake and I love the outdoors, and Blake was in his glory. He spent years reading adventure books, *Lost in the Barrens*, watching *Survivorman*, and hunting and fishing. Blake was waiting for the day to put his skills into practice in a real life survival situation where we weren't just pretending, we were in it!
>
> On the second day, Blake was feeling the lack of food. This trip just got real. I was content just eating rice, but Blake was convinced he needed meat in order to sustain himself. Then we saw one of the boys in the group coming down the trail holding what looked like a rope. He was singing, "...I'm coming home, I'm coming home, tell the world I'm coming home." *He's got a*

freaking snake in his hands! I thought. Blake was pumped! That's dinner. He paced with excitement. I remember thinking, *We are not eating this thing and I need to diffuse this right now,* but it was already a done deal in Blake's mind.

"Cameron, I hear what you're saying and I appreciate it," he said, "but I haven't eaten and I'm getting weak. I need protein to keep going, and I need to be able to hunt and provide for the group."

So we cooked the snake and ate it!

Recognizing what really mattered to Blake and encouraging him turned out to be an amazing experience. Blake knew it from the start! The whole group was impressed with Blake's skills and appreciated his patience, humour in the situation, and what he had to offer to the group.

Believe it or not, I ate it. It tasted like smoked salmon. All that was missing were the cheese and crackers!

At the end of the week, I finished with an Advanced Wilderness Survival Camp certificate and many new skills. This experience gave me strength to carry on in other difficult situations I would face in life. An added bonus was having another autistic person in a mentor role—it inspired me; when you have like-minded people in leadership roles, anything is possible!

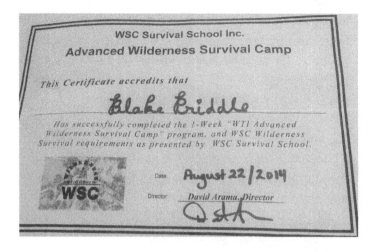

Certificate for my week-long survival camp

Travelling to new places far from home and going outside my comfort zone really prepared me for my future, and it built the confidence I needed to move far from home to get a job in the radio industry. I thank my parents for taking me on all these wonderful adventures and for pushing me to be independent. I hope to go on other adventures someday. My future travel list includes Norway, Grenada, Uganda, Japan, Madagascar and Paris. My next big adventure would be after I graduated from college.

Crushes and Dating

**"Always remember that even in darkness
you will always be loved
because your life is precious and should
not be taken for granted."**

Me

☆

My first exposure to dating occurred in Grade 7. Before the elementary school prom, I asked a girl I had a crush on to the prom dance. She was graduating elementary school and I had one more year. It was funny because Ms. Spry, my special education teacher, prompted me with what to say while the girl was standing there! I was so relieved that she said "yes," and I was really happy to have a date for the first time. Because she was in a wheelchair, she wasn't able to dance, so we sat and talked until the music got too loud for me. I was disappointed that I had to leave early because things didn't go as I had expected. I was really feeling the stress of a long night. The girl I went with understood and was still happy I had spent time with her at the dance.

The whole night wasn't bad. I had my first date, which was something to strike from my bucket list. I got some photos taken with her, and I was unexpectedly called up to the stage during the graduation ceremony to accept a citizenship award for being a good person and caring for others. Had I not had a date, I would have skipped the ceremony and missed the award presentation. This date helped me learn that dating isn't all sunshine and rainbows; sometimes it can involve disappointment and even heartbreak. Neither of us was heartbroken though, and we remained friends.

In Grade 8, I mustered my courage to try another date. Rather than being too forward, I told this person that I wasn't asking her to be my girlfriend, it was just a social outing (even though it would have been nice if we were actually dating). We went to a Halloween dance and slow danced together as friends. Later, we attended the Grade 8 graduation dance together where we had another slow dance. There was one girl there who couldn't find her date, so I offered to dance with her for a few songs after ensuring that my date was okay with this. We continued to be good friends throughout high school, but we never dated.

My parents told me there was no rush to have a girlfriend. Lots of people don't find girlfriends until after high school, and some people never do. It seemed like everyone at my school was dating, and it made me want a girlfriend even more. My parents bought me a book about dating for teenagers with Asperger's and it had some good tips on how I should dress, how to approach someone appropriately and when is a good time to have sex.

In June of 2012, just a few weeks before graduating high school, I had my first real dating relationship. We never got intimate, but we spent time together going fishing and to the senior prom. She asked me to the prom, which was flattering; a girl had never asked me out before! This gave me the impression that she was interested in me, and she was a good friend. We were originally going to go in a limo with some of her "friends," but when they found out I would be there they backed out. They thought I might call the police if they drank alcohol in the car. Her friends were being ignorant—I would never do that. Maybe they thought there'd be a repeat from the "Italian incident," but that was different because the teachers said the trip could be cancelled if the students drank on the trip. I guess they thought that because I was autistic, breaking the rules would drive me crazy. Of course, this was not true.

On the night of the prom, we had a dinner date at a local restaurant. It started off okay because driving to the prom and the restaurant seemed somewhat romantic in the town car that my parents rented for us. But when we got to the prom things went downhill. This prom wasn't organized by the school, and alcohol was served even though most of the students were underage. I was jealous that so many students had fake IDs and I didn't. I wanted to drink as well. To make matters worse, my friend didn't want to dance or do anything. She went home early complaining that her stomach was upset. Could this night get any worse? Luckily it didn't, as my cousin Steven and his girlfriend Veronica were visiting us at the time and my family friends Cam and Rachel were prom chaperones. The five of us went home and had a dance party in the basement, and I drank all the beer I wanted.

Spending the night with caring people was so much better than spending it with a date who didn't want to be with me. About a week later my friend sent me a text saying that she had found someone else and it was over. I was completely heartbroken at first, but my life coach Sandy helped me through it with a good pep talk. She recalled that this heartbreaking incident showed me who my true friends were. "It was difficult to see the disappointment Blake felt at the time, and even though he was really upset he offered me tea—always a perfect gentleman." She knew what it was like as she has three kids that have all been through breakups.

I learned a lot from these relationships, and I feel more comfortable living alone now. These relationships require too much commitment, as does having children. I like my space and privacy, and I also want to follow my own path. I feel these priorities would be affected in a relationship with a partner. Perhaps later on I'll change my mind, but for now I plan to stay celibate. My parents were right, there is no rush to find a relationship after all. Any future girlfriend or partner must be as supportive of my dreams as I would be of theirs.

The Car Crash or "Sh#* Happens"

I was eighteen and had been driving by myself for about three months when I got into a car crash on the highway. It was the day before the Easter long weekend, so traffic was heavy as I drove home from theatre rehearsal. When I arrived at the spot I normally turn left, I had to wait because there was a long line of cars heading my way. I looked behind to see if there were any cars coming, and sure enough there was a minivan bearing down on me—and it didn't look like it was slowing down. I knew a crash was imminent, so I braced myself and then, BANG! I was rear ended by the minivan going 80 km/hour. I was still conscious after the impact, but I was whiplashed and stunned, and I had hit my head on the headrest. I pulled to the side of the road and waited a few seconds before getting out. I figured my parents' new car was fixable, but the same could not be said about the other guy's vehicle. I walked over to them and, surprisingly, I didn't get angry as many people might have.

"Is everyone okay?" I asked.

Everyone was okay, except the guy's children were scared and crying. His mother had hurt herself on the seatbelt and his father's coffee had exploded all over himself. The driver seemed remorseful. He was relieved that his kids were okay. He had been distracted for just a few seconds to tell his kids to stop fighting in the back seat.

I was very shaken up by the accident, and I needed to talk to someone I trusted, so I called my neighbour Arielle. She had been t-boned at the same intersection, and I thought if anyone would know what do in this situation it would be her. She came right away when I told her what happened. A few minutes later, Arielle's dad Rob stopped to make sure I was okay. When the police arrived, they assessed the situation and the officer said that it clearly wasn't my fault, which made me feel better. The other guy had to have his car towed off the road since it was totalled. Even though my car was still driveable, I had Arielle give me a lift back to the house because I was too shaken up to drive. The police officer gave me the option of giving my statement the next day since she knew I was in shock.

I still felt the need to call my mom and dad to tell them what had happened, but since they were out of the country it was difficult to reach them. I needed reassurance because even though I knew I wasn't at fault, I was worried my parents would be mad at me over the damage to the car. This is what my parents recalled of the car crash calls. "We had been out of cell service during the day so when we checked our voicemail we had no less than fourteen increasingly frantic messages from Blake. Every parent's nightmare! But hearing his voice, however frantic, meant he was still okay! Knowing he had the Browns assisting him put us at ease as well."

Dawna and Rob advised me to go to the hospital to get checked out just in case I was injured, and it's a good thing that I did because my neck started to feel tender. My injuries were not overly serious, I just had to be careful not to strain my neck too much. As I waited for a doctor to assess me, I finally reached my parents on the phone and told them what had happened. They told me that they weren't upset with me at all and that even if the accident had been my fault, they still wouldn't have reprimanded me because they are called accidents for a reason. As for the car, Dad said, "It is just a car and it can be repaired." The important thing was that I was okay. I was so relieved to hear this from my parents.

Later that night, Mr. D called me and said the same as my mom and dad. He said not to worry about it because "shit happens." Having all this support made my situation bearable. When the officer came the next morning, the Browns came over as well and offered to help with my statement in case I needed clarification or something reworded.

Before I gave my statement, the officer informed us that the driver who ran into me was charged with careless driving.

After giving my statement, the Browns urged me to go for a drive. I was reluctant at first, but they said that when Arielle had been in her accident, she put off driving for a long time. They were worried that the more I put it off the longer it would be before I felt comfortable behind the wheel. I finally drove to the corner store to buy the Browns a thank you card for helping me through the ordeal.

The Browns said they were very impressed at how well I handled myself, and this made me proud. The trauma of the accident affected me for a while afterwards. You might say I had a mild form of Post Traumatic Stress Disorder (PTSD), and I had a difficult time turning at that intersection for months afterwards. Mr. D added some levity to the experience by nicknaming me "Crash" Priddle, something I took with good humour. I later took the name "Crash" as my radio stage name.

The best thing I got out of this experience was knowing how many people had supported me and how good they made me feel. Whenever I go through a tough time in my life and feel alone, I remember those who helped me in my time of need. I know there will always be someone who cares and wants to help. As Mr. Rogers said, "Always look for the people who are helping."

My First Job

It's really important for people on the spectrum to be employed in one way or another. I have seen parents on social media say their kids are unemployable. Temple Grandin, one of my heroes, used to clean horse stalls. Even if your kids can't work a minimum wage job, there are all kinds of things that autistic people can do. They can stuff envelopes, mow people's lawns or shovel snow. If they have other skills like painting or writing, they should use them!

In Grade 8, my mom got me involved in a program that helped teens on the autism spectrum prepare for the workforce. She had to take time off work to drive me seventy kilometres each week to the program, but she says it was worth it. It covered all the basic aspects of the workplace like what to do in a job interview, how to behave on the job and how to deal with customers properly. I found the program valuable, and it was well taught.

My first job didn't just happen. My mom was instrumental in helping create the supported employment program, and she fought for it to be offered in our community. She sat on the board of directors of the agency that offered the program and used that as leverage to bring the program to my town. It's another quiet example of her acting as my scaffold and advocate. Thankfully, there are more job training programs becoming available, but we still have a long way to go until all of us have meaningful and inclusive work, especially in rural and northern communities.

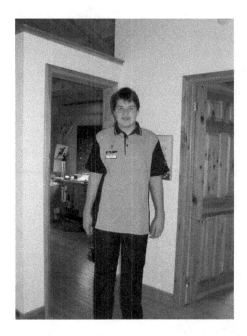

Me in my polyester grocery store uniform.
Wore it two times a week after school

I chose not to apply for a part-time job until Grade 9 because I wanted to have one last free summer before high school. I was fortunate to obtain a job at Winkel's, a grocery store in Espanola. The owners (whom my parents knew) understood I needed accommodations, and they did a great job meeting my needs. I was lucky that they were willing to give me only a couple of three-hour shifts a week since I was already overwhelmed with the duties of high school. I was called a front end service clerk, which is a fancy term for a janitor. I spent a good amount of my time cleaning and bringing in shopping carts.

My job mentor was very helpful during my first week of training. She was also an EA at my school, so she knew a thing or two about kids who are different. When she taught me how to call someone over the store intercom, she was impressed at how well I managed to make the page. She told me she was nervous the first time she had done it, so I felt proud that I was able to do something other workers couldn't do comfortably. You could say that it was my first taste of professional radio! One time I had to make the announcement that the store was closing because the cashiers were too scared to do it themselves. They were all impressed by how I made the announcement and said I should be in radio.

My "pocketbook"—a special book my job coaches made for me—really helped with the Winkel's job. It contained all the step-by-step instructions for my job, so if I forgot what I was supposed to do, I would simply refer to the pocketbook. It helped that the instructions were listed in the proper order with pictures and words; it was perfectly organized. Anyone can use a pocketbook on their new job, not just those on the spectrum. After about a month or so, I was so used to the routine that I no longer needed it, but it really came in handy during the early days.

Things went well over the three years I worked at Winkel's. I only recall dealing with one rude customer. I was asked to help load some bags of manure into a customer's car, and due to a miscommunication, I thought I was just supposed to put in one bag not eight. So, after I had loaded one, he stood by his car waiting. I couldn't figure out why he wasn't leaving, so we kind of awkwardly stared at each other. He ended up loading the rest of the bags by himself and then he got upset with me and was very rude. I told my job mentor what happened, and she said I'd come across people in the workplace who are rude from time to time. She knew how it felt because she had dealt with rude customers before as well.

The owners and supervisors liked me because of my efficiency. At the end of my shift I always called the supervisor to ask if there was anything else I could do before I punched out. On my last day at Winkel's, I gave the two owners a thank you card telling them how appreciative I was. This first job helped prepare me for the work force.

Realizing My Passion: First Steps in Media

Even as a child I knew I wanted to have some form of career in media, anything from news reporter to actor or radio personality. I loved listening to the local radio stations in the car and at home, and I liked hearing the personalities talk back and forth. It sounded like they were having fun and this made me want to work in radio and entertain people the same way. Sometimes I would pretend I was a news anchor and make up my own news stories and Mom would pretend to watch me on TV. I was also interested in newspaper journalism. One of my respite workers was a freelance writer, which I thought was a cool, and she inspired me to write for a newspaper one day.

Working as an actor in movies and TV shows appealed to me, but my parents warned me it is difficult to get a job in that field. I had other ideas for a career as I grew up, and I really didn't consider working in media seriously until Grade 8. Before attending high school, I visited the CTV station in Sudbury with the Autism March Break camp I attended, and my interest was piqued!

As luck would have it, EHS had a program called Spartan Youth Radio (SYR), a media club that specialized in podcasts and videos. When I first heard about the program, I knew I would be a part of it throughout my time in high school. I had the pleasure of being mentored by Jayson Stewart, a.k.a. Mister Stew. Mister Stew wrote about the time I spent at Spartan Youth Radio with him:

> I ran Spartan Youth Radio, Canada's first high school podcast radio station. Over time, it morphed into a multi-media journalism program where the students created audio, video and written news stories, rants, opinion pieces and culture reviews. But we were best

known for our interviews of heavy-hitting celebrities. I was working alone in the studio one day with the door open. The lighting was subdued, I'm sure I had music on, and I was either editing content or arranging some upcoming production when Blake was brought in to meet me as part of his personal tour of the school.

I first noticed that he was exceptionally gregarious and full of questions about the type of music we played, what we did and how he could be involved. His eyes were darting all over the room, he was nearly vibrating with energy and, at first, I thought he was asking questions and then tuning me out, but I soon realized he was absorbing EVERYTHING. By the end of the short visit, he was almost salivating at the thought of joining the program in Grade 9. Later that day, Mr. Diebel came in to visit and tell me more about Blake and his skills, challenges and the plans for the coming entry into Grade 9.

During the first week of September as we were launching our next season of Spartan Youth Radio, Blake came in and was bouncing off the walls, excited for all the music he was going to play and the interviews he was going to conduct.

At one of our first meetings, I challenged the reporters to come up with a list of people they would like to interview or stories they would like to cover. Blake asked if there was a limit to who he could put on his list.

"Other than them being alive, put anyone on there that you would like to chat with," I said. "Many will say no, most will ignore us, but a few might say yes, and we run with those."

He had a number of names on his list including Stuart McLean, Crystal Shawanda and Les Stroud. Within two years, Blake had interviewed all three and many more.

Every time there was an SYR field trip, Blake was there. Every time there was a meeting, Blake was there. Every time there was food, Blake was there! Even when Blake was not at the school, like when he travelled through Europe, SYR wasn't far from Blake's mind. One of my cherished set of photos are of the SYR logo held up selfie-style in monuments across the US and Europe that Blake was visiting.

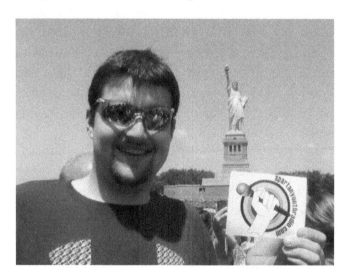

Checking out the Statue of Liberty

What did I notice that was different about Blake? Everything. And nothing. He was a teenager who wanted to be loved, wanted to catch the attention of the right girl, wanted to do well in school, wanted to bag the biggest buck or catch the biggest fish. But Blake was and is so much more than that.

I noticed in him a passion for a world that often confused him. I saw him go through mental breakdowns where he misinterpreted what someone said, missed out on someone's body language or was misinterpreted or misunderstood himself. There was a time where he quit Spartan Youth Radio altogether because of one of these misinterpretations. I remember being the cause or the perceived cause of some offence that sent Blake to Resource to take a week or so and come back to his old haunts in the SYR studio.

When I heard Blake was pursuing radio broadcasting, I was elated. I knew he would be good at it and would make a name for himself. Even if it was a short-term career, I knew that spending time in the real world and working with a broadcasting team would be good for him, for his maturity, for his growth and sense of empowerment. It's an honour to have had him in my program, to consider him a friend and to see his growth in so many different ways. Go Blake! Like Spartan Youth Radio, you're "all kinds of different," and we celebrate that!

It was the thought of interviewing famous people as well as the encouragement from my teachers and my parents that made me want to try something new. Mom and Dad told me that if I wanted to pursue a career in media, it would be best to get as much experience as possible, and I would have more knowledge of the field if I joined SYR.

I quit going to SYR in the second semester of Grade 9 because I didn't feel like I fit in. I had trouble accepting how the older members ran the place, and I realized it really wasn't a "radio station." In Grade 10, I decided to give SYR a second chance, and did it ever pay off! I learned that SYR wasn't what I thought it would be. But nothing really ever is! One of the things that changed was that the club now had a music licence so we could play whatever music we wanted without legal problems. Also, I was able to interview people for the first time.

The other thing that changed was the attitude the other members had toward me. They were more positive, and I felt more a part of the group than I had in Grade 9.

Most newcomers to media don't interview people who are famous, but my first ever interview was with Les Stroud, better known to his fans from the show *Survivorman*. We managed to get in touch with him through a few family connections, and my interview with Les became a reality—something I had always wanted to do. To this day, it is one of my most memorable interviews even though I had no prior interviewing experience and was only fifteen at the time.

I also had the pleasure of interviewing country music singer Crystal Shawanda twice during my time with SYR. Once I caught some momentum, I sat down with country singer Larry Berrio, my cousin Steven Beyers who played hockey in the OHL, sportscaster Dave Hodge, and Stuart McLean, the former host of *The Vinyl Café* radio show. The in-person interview with Stuart McLean was special because I learned that we had a lot in common. He told me he was very shy as a child but he still managed to have an amazing career in radio and made so many people laugh with his stories. Stuart passed away a few years ago, and it was really hard on me because often when you interview someone you get to know them and you make a friend in just a few minutes. Getting to meet him was an opportunity of a lifetime.

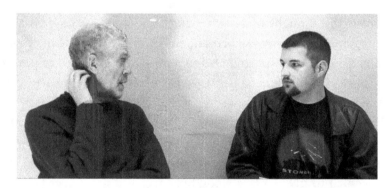

Amazing highlight: meeting and interviewing the iconic Stuart McLean

In Grade 11, I tried to determine whether I should pursue a career in television or radio. In SYR, I produced podcast interviews, podcast radio music shows and video interviews, so I had diverse experience. I decided to pursue radio because I felt I stood a better chance of hosting my own show, which was something I really wanted to do. I needed to gain experience in a real radio station, so I applied for a co-operative education placement at the local commercial station. As luck would have it, I landed a half-day placement with the morning show host, probably the best possible scenario. The host was very friendly and understanding of my needs. I learned the procedure of hosting a show, how a radio station works and how radio commercials are made. The best part was getting to co-host and have a few laughs on the morning show. I also got to voice the weather and the community events.

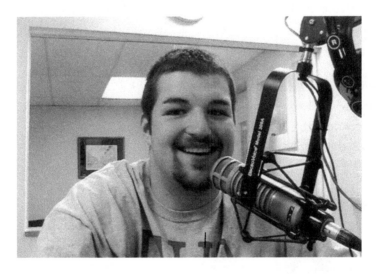

First time on radio. My high school co-op placement, Moose FM, Espanola

If Mister Stew hadn't encouraged me to try SYR again, I probably wouldn't have taken that co-op placement which helped my career in media so much. I wrote and conducted all those interviews, produced all those podcast radio shows and contributed as much as I could. I worked so hard that I won SYR Employee of the Year in Grade 12. I just can't thank Mister Stew enough for giving me a chance to be part of the team at SYR, and the local radio station in Espanola for giving me a co-op placement.

After graduating high school, I worked the summer at the local newspaper, *The Mid North Monitor*, as a freelance journalist. I was mentored by a compassionate editor, Rosalind (Roz) Russell, who, besides having radio experience, had lots of patience to show me the ropes. Roz recalled:

> When Blake was stressed, he tumbled his words. It was just a matter of telling him to stop, breathe and take time. It helped Blake find his composure. I found Blake would not always look at me eye-to-eye or would do so intensely depending on the discussion we were having. Blake took time before responding. I could see him organizing his thoughts before he vocalized them—he is a methodical thinker, which is a good thing.

Working at SYR, the newspaper and 99.3 Moose FM helped me prepare for the next step of my media career at Loyalist College in the radio broadcasting program. So off I went—making my parents empty-nesters—transitioning to college and adulthood.

Chapter 4:

Adulthood 101

Time to Do My Own Laundry

I had dreamt about going to college ever since I started high school. I was eager to take a course that would help me prepare for my dream career, and I wanted some independence. Mom and Dad were reluctant to allow me to go away at first because they were unsure if I was ready to manage at a new school in a new city. They thought it would be beneficial if I spent a year taking a general arts and science course at Cambrian College closer to home. I did not agree as I didn't want to waste a whole year studying something I wasn't interested in.

I researched all kinds of radio broadcasting courses. The best match seemed to be Loyalist College in Belleville, Ontario. Mom liked it because it was a campus in a smaller city, and she believed I stood a better chance of getting the help I needed from my professors. We arranged to tour the college and quickly learned that it was a great course and the college had all the amenities a student could need. We also found out that the program was open to learning disabled students. I felt this was the place for me, but my mom was still worried about how well I would do with a full course load. She had fought hard for me to get the accommodations I needed in high school, which I appreciated, but I felt that if I could overcome the challenges I faced in high school, with or without certain accommodations, then I could handle the challenges of college.

I was accepted into the radio broadcasting program and, although I registered for a full course load, I had the option for a reduced load if I felt I needed it. In the summer of 2012, I took another campus tour to check out residence where I would be staying for the following two years. The common area had a laundry room, table games and a nice living room-like area with a fireplace where we could study. This made me feel right at home. I also learned about the weekly pool tournaments, sundae bars and bingo. It was amazing just how much stuff they had to offer.

Away I Went: The time to go to college came at last at the end of August. Leaving home was extremely nerve-wracking. I was taking my first real step into adulthood and moving eight hours away. I was excited as well because I knew I would be doing something I liked. After not sleeping well, the first day of college was finally here.

Meeting my roommates on the first day helped ease my angst. Orientation involved the professors introducing themselves and making us all feel welcome. I met some of my classmates and we shared our media experience. I mentioned the people I interviewed in high school, and my classmates seemed impressed.

The first few weeks of classes went pretty smoothly, and I was getting along well with my roommates, but the courses soon became more challenging. I did okay at writing commercials since I had a bit of experience, but there were other things I wasn't prepared for. One of the biggest challenges was the announcing techniques course. I had no idea what to do even though I had been on the radio before. The show prep had been done for me, and my radio voice wasn't the problem either; it was my lack of preparation skills that failed me.

First Taste of Frank Feedback: After hosting a couple of horrible shifts on Hot Hits (the school's radio station), I had the unpleasant task of showing my breaks (what the announcer says in between songs) to my professor. I quickly learned that this guy didn't mince words when it came to criticism! He never said anything to my face, but on the class website he wrote things like: "The entire break was awful and unprepared," and, "Joke very lame, if you're not funny don't try to be." I had never been criticized in such a brutally honest way before. I was furious to the point where I showed the messages to my parents in disbelief. I really disliked this professor because of his criticism, but my parents encouraged me to not take his comments personally and instead use them to do better.

As I look back now, I feel that had it not been for the frank criticism I wouldn't be the person I am today, and I never would have developed the thick skin I need to work in the media. This program pushed me to work harder than even before so I could impress my professors and improve my skills.

Toward the end of the year, I finally managed to get full marks on a commercial assignment where we had to produce a commercial about an Easter egg hunt. My professor said it was well-written and produced.

I was happy I had finally produced a radio ad he loved and gave me full marks for, as I was beginning to doubt that I could.

My other big accomplishment was my audio documentary on Michael Jackson. I worked long hours on this project and earned full marks for it.

Disclose or Not?

I first disclosed my autism to my professors in the second semester. We had a big test toward the end of the first year. I had studied hard for it, but the questions were written in a way I didn't understand. I handed the test in without writing much on it. This was really embarrassing as I am not a quitter, but I didn't know what to do. My mom encouraged me to explain my situation to the professor and ask if she could rephrase the questions in an oral format.

I met with my professor and explained that I have high functioning autism and sometimes needed certain elements to be rephrased. She didn't hesitate for a second and had no problem allowing me to do the test orally. She read the questions to me again and then rephrased so I would understand and earn the passing grade I deserved.

Social Scene

The first semester went by really fast, but college is more than just doing work and going to classes—there has to be social life as well. Loyalist College had a social group for people on the autism spectrum, but I chose not to get involved. I thought it would be better to spend time with *typical* people and not rely on autism groups to make friends. I really didn't have a lot in common with this group because they weren't interested in partying or anything that I was interested in—or so I thought.

I was social with my classmates, and I would try to make small talk whenever I could. We didn't do much together outside of school. We all got along well, and they were really nice to me. Some of them were around my age, but a lot of them were in their 30s or 40s. I remember hanging out with two of my classmates one day on a break and we went behind a bush to smoke some pot, something I had never done before. They were patient with me and didn't force me to try it. Right then and there, I knew I could trust these guys. I chose to take a puff because I was curious about what weed would do to me and what it feels like to get high. I took the occasional toke during my years at college, and one time I got so high I fell right to sleep. Another one of my classmates gave me some tips on where to get cannabis and how to use it responsibly.

Although it's good to be social, sometimes I needed time for myself, and I spent a lot of time alone. I would often go see a movie on the weekend and write a short review of it so I could have something to talk about when I did a talk break on the radio at school. There were times when I felt homesick for my family and friends back home, and I sometimes felt like I didn't fit in in southern Ontario. I am a northerner at heart, and I didn't meet any people who liked to hunt and fish like I do.

Summer Radio Experience

I heaved a big sigh of relief when my first college year ended. I could finally take a break from assignments and focus on getting some real radio experience. Fortunately, with the help of an employment support program for people with disabilities run through the YMCA, I was able to secure a summer job at the radio station on Manitoulin Island. The job developer who found me the position cautioned my mom that this particular workplace was very laid-back and thus appeared disorganized. She worried that it wouldn't be suitable for someone on the spectrum since autistic people often have a difficult time with chaos and disorganization. My mom laughed and said I may be autistic but I am extremely disorganized and couldn't care less if things "weren't in order."

I was hired, and I quickly learned that this was going to be a fun place to work because the staff was very welcoming and friendly. The co-owner was a fantastic mentor. Within a week I was writing, voicing and producing commercials, and I announced the Community Happenings segment. I really enjoyed having the creative opportunity to produce radio ads that aired on the radio. A highlight of this summer position was the opportunity to host my own Canada Day show featuring famous Canadian country artists I'd interviewed in the past. I am thankful that they allowed me to get this kind of experience. The only thing I had a difficult time with was helping set up the Manitoulin Country Fest. While I enjoy concerts, I can't handle the heat so that was a hard grind. If only the festival was in the winter!

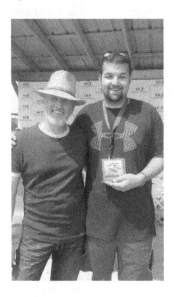

Meeting musician Kevin Closs at Manitoulin Country Fest

Round Two of College

**"It takes a stronger person to admit their
faults and accept the consequences than it is to
deny it and blame it on someone else."**

Me

☆

Summer went by quickly, as it always does, and it was time to start my second year at Loyalist. Little did I know that the first semester of the second year would be a tremendous test of my sanity and anxiety levels. We received a lot more homework than in first year, and this didn't give us a lot of free time to do anything social. I also had to deal with some new and unruly roommates, which was a real challenge.

Not everything about this semester was bad; I was finally allowed to do an on-air shift on the college's station, 91X, once or twice a week and host the station's all request show every now and then.

One day I felt so overwhelmed I suffered a minor panic attack. All students were required to take part in a certain number of promotional appearances in order to pass the semester. I had signed up to represent the campus station at a Halloween function. At the same time, we had a tough assignment to complete. The stress caused me to break down during a meeting at the studio. One of my teachers saw this and explained to the rest of the class what I was going through, and that he knew what a panic attack looked and felt like because he'd had them as well. He reminded me that panic attacks are no one's fault—they are just like coughs and sneezes, he said—and no one has complete control over them. This was so helpful to me and important for others in the class to hear.

After one stressful day at school, I came home completely overwhelmed. I felt sick to my stomach, had no energy and was in no mood to deal with my childish roommates. I was just about to fall asleep when one of my roommates started yelling about my ice cream container falling out of the freezer. I blew a fuse! I knew I should have just ignored him, but I completely lost it and we got into a full-blown argument. Before the verbal exchange had even started, someone tried to explain that my roommate was drunk, but I ignored her and the verbal fight continued.

My legs started to shake, and I knew if I didn't leave to walk it off I would lose it even more. After I left to cool off, I collapsed and had a full-blown panic attack at the bottom of the stairs. This was one of the worst panic attacks I have ever had. Some nursing students who were partying nearby noticed this and came to help. It was so bad that I didn't even know where I was, but I pointed to my medical alert bracelet. They took the keys off my neck to go to my room and get my wallet card that gave instructions on how to deal with my panic attacks and called 911 for help. When the paramedics came, they brought a gurney and checked my blood pressure. It felt like I was being treated like a heart attack patient, which was fitting because it really did feel like I was dying! At the hospital, I told the doctor exactly what had happened. He eventually sent me home with medication I could take if I ever felt another panic attack coming on.

My parents were travelling, so there was no way I could communicate with them that night. I did leave a bunch of messages which alarmed my mom. This is what she recalled:

> I checked my messages and saw nine missed calls from Blake. My heart sank with worry. Each call was more frantic until the last call that ended with his voice sounding so weary—no doubt the exhaustion brought on by the panic attack and the night's events. We were helpless being so far away, but we had set up a few safe people who could support Blake if things got worse.

I was afraid to go back to the dorm out of fear that my roommate might yell at me and possibly attack me. However, I heard him throwing up when I got home. *Serves him right!* I thought. I made myself a cup of herbal tea to sooth me to sleep, and it worked way better than any alcoholic beverage could. The next day I apologized for yelling at him, but he told me it was his fault and he was the one who should be sorry. Maybe he wasn't that bad after all.

About a week later I went to a Santa Clause parade out of town, and on the way back I got into an argument with one of my classmates. We were both stressed, and we spoke to one another in a way we wouldn't have had we been calm. Once I got out of the car I was in panic mode, hyperventilating, and I punched a sign to let out my anger. I apologized to the classmate, but just when I thought things couldn't get any worse, they did.

I was called into the office of the course co-ordinator—I knew this meant bad news. She told me she was really upset about the behaviour I had been exhibiting lately. She had heard that during one of my promotion appearances I had said some bad words while angry, and someone had been offended and complained. She told me that my behaviour was unacceptable and if I didn't change, I wouldn't be allowed to go into the community for my internship and would have to do it at the college radio station instead.

With all this going on, I had another panic attack right there in the co-ordinator's office. She tried to calm me down, but I couldn't. I woke up in the nurse's office after having calmed down a little, and I explained my issues. I phoned my mom and told her everything the professor said and how ashamed I felt. Although my mom assured me that doing an internship at the school's radio station wasn't a bad thing, I disagreed. I needed to be just like everyone else and go outside my comfort zone and do an internship outside of school.

I think the nurse told the rest of my professors that I was autistic. They had no idea because I was reluctant to tell them; I just wanted to be seen as "normal." I had come a long way in handling the challenging parts of my autism but clearly not far enough. I still needed help. Once they found out that I was autistic, they understood my behaviour more. They knew I wasn't a bad person but was just acting out because I was overwhelmed and stressed. I needed to learn more constructive ways to manage my anger and stress.

One of the professors said that if I ever felt overwhelmed or stressed to let him know. He said I could break a piece of Styrofoam he had laying around in his office to release my stress and my anger in a good way. With my autism disclosure, my professors had a much better understanding of my needs.

The third semester was one of the most difficult and stressful times of my life. You couldn't pay me to go through it again. At times I wanted to take a reduced course load, but I pushed through and passed with good marks. I was never happier to go home for Christmas break!

The final semester flew by. My attitude and overall motivation changed completely. Since I was not as stressed, I didn't have any panic attacks, punch signs or intimidate people. My professors noticed this as well, so I was allowed to go on my internship in Wawa to cap off the program.

College Internship

"The thing that's really great about doing a morning radio show is seeing the sunrise. A natural beauty that's not commonly seen by people who are not early risers. Somehow the feeling of a cup of coffee while watching the sunrise makes you feel like your soul is replenished after a night's rest. Ready to take on the day."

Me

☆

Wawa, a town in northern Ontario, is the setting of a movie called *Snow Cake* starring Sigourney Weaver and Alan Rickman. It is about a woman with autism. While I was there, I got to see some of the locations where the movie was filmed. If you haven't seen it, you need to because it's very heartwarming and inspirational.

The next chapter of my college experience, the internship, was mostly positive. I was working in a place where I knew I would feel at home, and I would be staying with close family friends. I was a little nervous about my first day at the station, like anyone would be. I knew what to expect, but my biggest fear was sleeping in because I had to be there for 5:00 a.m. Fortunately, I woke up without issue at 4:15 a.m. It took about fifteen minutes to walk to the station—imagine seeing the northern lights on your daily commute!

The owner said I would be doing a little bit of everything in my internship: operating the board, voice tracking and hosting. This is a rarity in most radio station internships. Since I had the opportunity to host, I was able to get some voice clips put together to add to my demo tape, which helped build my portfolio. The owner and the announcer were great mentors and were impressed with my effort.

I am grateful for this opportunity in Wawa which got me more extensive radio experience than my classmates. When I wasn't working, I went fishing with my friends Jami and Rob. One day, Rob, who is a helicopter pilot, flew me up to a lake to go fishing. One of my professors heard this and commented that not many students get to go heli-fishing on their internship!

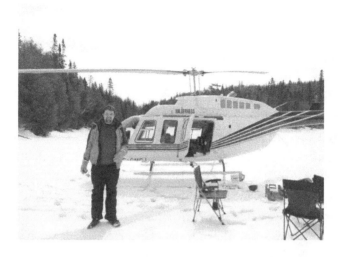

I'm likely the only one heli-fishing while on my college internship! *(courtesy J. Burns)*

Insights from One of My Cool Professors

The two years I spent at college played a big part of how I became the wiser person I am today.

I am going to let Craig Jackman, one of my professors, tell you about his experience with me in the radio broadcasting program:

> Blake was the first student I taught who identified on the autism spectrum. What I noticed is probably the same as everyone else: he was a nice young man who didn't like to make eye contact. His voice pattern was usually very even, detached being the wrong word. Even then it wasn't something that unusual from a lot of other students and just seemed a little socially awkward.
>
> For example, some things that would get a laugh from the class wouldn't get a reaction as much from Blake, and some things that the group didn't react to, Blake

did. I wouldn't say that's universal, but the occasional comment would have Blake laughing when nobody else was.

There were a few occasions of meltdown. One was in a professor's office that was severe enough to get health people involved, and I was only aware of it after the fact. The other showed more of the character of Blake's peers than any fault in him. I came into the room for a station ops meeting. Everyone in his group was in the room with Blake, close, but not too close. They told me Blake was having a bad day and that they were going to cancel my meeting until he got through what the problem was. There was no mocking, no false concern; they just wanted Blake to feel better. While it wasn't a normal day, they didn't let on that it was anything out of the ordinary, and they just kept everything calm.

Previously, I had thought of autism as an on/off issue. You were or you weren't. If you had autism you were non-functional and non-communicative. It was an educational experience for me as I didn't know that Blake could be autistic and highly functional, especially in the communications business.

I have learned that a student on the autism spectrum generally likes to do things in order—1-2-3-4—so I can see why news is an area of the business Blake can be successful in. Other spectrum students are the same. They like to follow an order or a pattern and gravitate to areas that will make them successful. That doesn't mean autism spectrum students aren't good at being spontaneous and creative. "We always do it that way, so let's do something different" must be a phrase that strikes fear into those kinds of students, and it's exactly the way I try and do things and get students to try. That doesn't mean they can't and don't put together beautiful and exciting sounding productions, they can and do; it's a difficult and learned behaviour that would be hard to develop and display over two academic years.

The last thing I'd like to add is that every year the faculty get together to argue about who should win what awards. Everyone has their favourite, and there is trading and discussion going back and forth. If your X student wins this award, then I think Y student has to get a different award. It's not a heated discussion, and in the end those who are deserving are rewarded and recognized. In Blake's case, it was Sandi who suggested that Blake be the faculty choice winner because of his dedication, effort and for overcoming obstacles. The response was unanimous in agreement. It was the right choice for the right reasons.

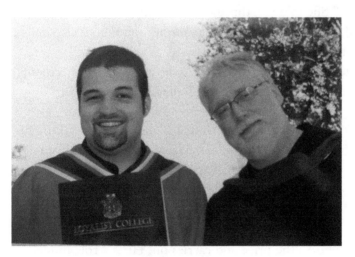

Me and one cool professor, C. Jackman, Loyalist College graduation, 2014

Graduation!

I found out I won the faculty choice award about a month after my internship. I also found out I made the Dean's List with an average

80.05%. Mom and Dad revealed my final score by giving me a congratulations card with eighty dollars and five cents. I was really proud of both these accomplishments; it was proof that my hard worked paid off and being through hell and back at times was worth it. At first, I didn't know why or how I was chosen for the award because I acted out under stress in an unprofessional manner a few times. Mom told me I managed to overcome all those challenges and I didn't give up; I fought until the end to succeed. She thought I showed my professors that I learned from mistakes and was committed to the course and the radio industry.

My graduation ceremony was in June, and I was surrounded by supportive friends, family, professors and peers. After the ceremony, I met with Sandi Ramsay, the professor who nominated me for the faculty choice award. She said some very kind things about me. "It was a privilege to share in Blake's post-secondary learning journey. Watching him grow, striving to achieve and making it happen! His personality is infectious, that's why so many of Blake's peers shared fondness for him too." She told me, through tears of joy, that I was an inspiration to her and I helped to give her hope for her son who is also on the autism spectrum.

A dear family friend, Marie T., who attended my ceremony, recalled my time in college and being in Belleville for two years:

> I was very glad to learn that Blake would be taking his media studies course in the same town where I lived. He was generous of spirit and willing to hang out with an "old" lady for a couple of dinners out. It was fun. I was so proud of him, his courage and determination. Blake knows what it costs to fall down and get up again, but he pays the price and carries on. He is a role model. It was a privilege for me to be invited to his graduation, and I cried with joy.

A simple message I have for parents with autistic children attending school or post-secondary school: things will seem bad at times as we learn and grow, but it does gets better.

Got the Diploma, Now What?

Once I finished college it was time to find a full-time job in my field. I really underestimated just how difficult that would be. I had assumed that if I had a college diploma, I would get a job in my field easily. I was wrong. It was the classic dilemma: I couldn't get a job because I didn't have enough experience, and I couldn't get more experience without a job. So I decided to do what was needed to build my resume and industry skills while fine-tuning my life skills.

Island Radio—The Kick-Starter: Fortunately, the owners of the radio station on Manitoulin Island agreed to have me work in a part-time limited contract position. I was happy to have the opportunity to work at the Island station again because I had had a blast working for them the previous summer. Since I was only working part-time, I also applied for full-time radio jobs whenever I could.

Island Radio presented a new set of challenges and opportunities. I filled in for the afternoon host whenever he was unavailable and was very excited to host my own weekly pre-recorded volunteer show which I called "Crash's Campfire." It seemed really cool at the time, but I look back on it now and realize it wasn't my greatest effort.

After airing one of the first episodes of the show, I learned the importance of being more vigilant and double-checking content before putting it on the air. I had found a song online that I thought sounded like a good campfire song, but I didn't bother to listen to the whole song. I played it on the show not knowing that it contained some lyrics that were inappropriate and offensive for public radio. When I realized this, I was frozen with fear and didn't know what would happen to me next. Would I get fired? Would I be thought of poorly by the public? It was more than I could bear, and I broke down and had a panic attack. In between breaths I managed to tell my boss what happened. She assured me I wasn't going to get fired and the worst-case scenario was they would need to do some damage control but nothing more. I had been so excited about hosting and airing my own show and I had messed up. I was too excited and didn't think about what I was putting on the air. This experience was not in vain. It made me a wiser person and a better broadcaster. Ever since then, I have always listened to all content that I plan to put on the air.

I didn't get hired at the end of my contract, but they were supportive in allowing me to volunteer twice a week. I owe a lot to the owner who was also a great mentor. This experience kick-started my career in radio.

We All Need a Life Coach at Times

During that fall, my mom lined up a grant to offset the cost for a life coach, Theresa Laurenti, on certain days after work. I was wary of the idea at first and didn't think I needed a coach, but working with Theresa was one of the best things to happen to me! It was like having Sharon Sproule as a mentor, but we didn't just focus on theatre. We also practised writing, improv, and I even took some music lessons.

Theresa recommended I make myself known as much as possible and suggested I start a Facebook page so people could follow me and keep up to date with what I was doing. She helped me organize my resume and applications for jobs. None of them ever got back to me, but it was good experience.

I knew that if I was going to work in radio it was important to connect with people in the community so they could get to know me and I could attract new listeners. The local Lions Club held TV bingo every Wednesday night, and I thought that if I joined the Lions Club, I could practise my on-air skills on the local TV station and give back to the community at the same time.

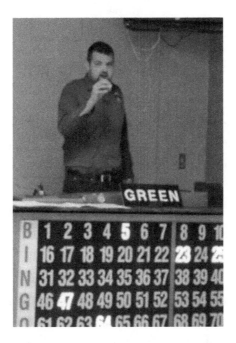

Calling Lions Club TV bingo, Espanola, ON

It wasn't long before I started to call bingo for the Lions Club on the local cable TV station. This was my first taste of live TV, but I wasn't overly nervous. With the exception of the audience being able to see me, it wasn't much different than live radio. In between games I announced upcoming community events, which was a good opportunity to practise reading on air.

One of the more memorable moments of being a Lion was meeting Carol Hughes, our member of parliament (MP), at a seniors' supper the Lions organized as part of Espanola's winter carnival. On Theresa's advice, I used this opportunity to practise my interviewing skills. I took a digital recorder along and hoped to interview some people at the dinner and turn it into a news story/podcast for my new Facebook page. Carol gave a short speech and praised me for the work I was doing with the Lions Club. She said it was such a good thing to have young people like me volunteering to make a difference. Being praised by a politician for my work was an amazing feeling.

One of the longtime Lions members, Dario, shared his thoughts about my time in the Lions Club:

When Blake joined the club, I don't think many Lions members knew he was autistic. He was just a nice individual who wanted to help. As a matter of fact, we were so happy he joined because he was a young member with many ideas to share. This gave us a new perspective when it came to the younger generation, as most of our members are retired. We welcomed his position on many items brought up in the agenda.

I remember him serving hot dogs and juice boxes to the many kids who attended the children's Christmas party. He always had a smile on his face and welcomed everyone.

The seniors' supper also benefitted from Blake's help. This project is so massive that it takes our whole club to bring it about. Blake was popular with the seniors since he was well-known for his drama performances and presence in the community.

Having autism never hindered him from contributing to the club and its functions. When he left Espanola for a job up north, we missed him, but he came back to add his input until going off again to pursue his career. We would welcome Blake back to our club any time.

Around this time, I started to volunteer at Sacred Heart Elementary School in Espanola with Theresa. Our family friend, Shelley (who was the special ed teacher there), told us there was a boy at the school, Spencer, who was on the autism spectrum and that it would be good if someone could do some social skills work with him twice a week. Spencer's sister was playing Alice in the school production of *Alice in Wonderland*, and that meant I could do some work with the kids in the school play as well.

I first met Spencer in January of 2015. He recognized me from another community autism event we had both attended when he was in kindergarten. I was amazed at how good his memory was! I saw a lot of myself in Spencer; I first noticed that his voice was naturally projected, and he often had trouble using an inside voice. I, too, had struggled with that as a child.

I experienced all kinds of teachable moments and faced many difficulties over the years, and this made working with Spencer easy because I could pass knowledge to him. We played turn-taking games and worked on social skills and how to deal with difficult situations properly without making other people uncomfortable. I even thought outside the box and bought a Social Stories board game which offered Spencer and some of the other kids the opportunity to tell their stories. I think Spencer really enjoyed working with me, as his mother told me he would often talk at the dinner table about how much fun I was to be with. I know it would have helped me to have an older mentor who was also autistic.

School was sometimes difficult for Spencer because it wasn't easy to make friends and some of his peers didn't know how to interact with him because he was different. Theresa and I decided to do a special presentation about inclusion and acceptance for all of Spencer's classmates as well as some students in other classes. The kids really enjoyed the presentation, and it gave me the opportunity to tell my story as well. The school board made a YouTube video of this experience.

I also had the pleasure of working as an assistant director for the school play. I had always wanted to direct a play, and this gave me the opportunity to be a little bit like Sharon Sproule, my theatre mentor. I helped the actors work on their lines, but if they messed up or if I saw them playing with their sleeves or if they weren't loud enough, I would make them start over. They seemed puzzled by this, so I explained that we had to practise until each move was right—it is how it's done in theatre. It was funny that I was teaching these students to use a big voice because we were working with Spencer to use his inside voice.

Out of all the things I taught these students, the most important was responsibility. They needed to learn their lines and be prepared so they didn't let others down.

Theresa and I worked on recognizing other people's emotions as well. One day we went to the mall to observe people's facial expressions and the way they walked. We then discussed how they might be feeling. It was really fun, and I used some of what she taught me when I worked with Spencer. Here were her tips:

- Since managing our emotions is one of the biggest hurdles for all of us, and particularly challenging for most people with autism, learning how the body responds to thoughts is essential.
- Thoughts trigger emotions.
- Emotions dictate our language and actions.
- Language and actions further trigger emotions.
- Reversing the situation so you can put yourself in someone else's shoes can sometimes help you discover a new perspective.

Another way I volunteered in the community was to act as a contributor to the local Autism Acceptance group. On World Autism Awareness Day, I was interviewed on CBC Radio's *Morning North* with one of my job coaches from the YMCA to talk about employment and my experiences with autism. That same day I attended an autism flag raising ceremony in front of the town hall in Espanola with the Autism Acceptance group.

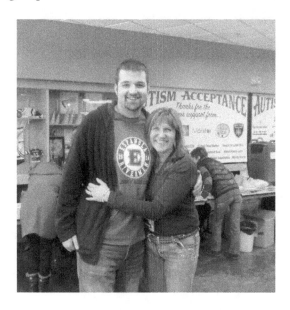

My amazing life coach, Theresa

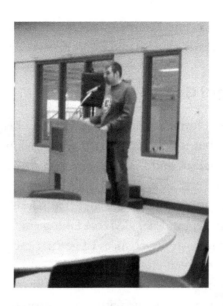

**Telling a bit of my life story at our local Autism
Acceptance event, Espanola, Ontario**

My friend Dennis Lendrum started the local Autism Acceptance group. He organized many events and began advocating for better services and inclusion after his grandson was diagnosed. One time he arranged for autistic children and their families to meet with local law enforcement and fire fighters so they could get to know each other and share more about autism. At one of these family events, I was asked to tell people my story. The speech was well-received, especially by those on the spectrum and their parents. This event was so much fun, and the best part was having country music singer Crystal Shawanda attend. It was awesome to find out she supported the autism community.

Another opportunity arose for me to practise my interpersonal and sales skills when our family friend Leigh McAdam had a new book published. It was about hiking and other adventures that people can do across Canada, and it needed to be distributed in northern Ontario since there were a lot of attractions from that region featured in her book. I made a list of stores I thought would be interested in selling copies. While many places came to mind, I knew that with sales and marketing people won't always say yes, so Mom helped me put together a sales script. I found a fair number of stores that were willing to sell the books, and Leigh really appreciated my initiative.

Back to College I Go

Doing all this volunteer work and distributing Leigh's book helped build my resume, but it wasn't paying the bills. Mom told me about a postgraduate journalism and news reporting course at Seneca College in Toronto. Paula Todd, a well-known Canadian journalist, was one of the professors. I wasn't sure about it at first because I aimed to get a job right after college, but I decided that taking another course to build my skills would improve my chances of getting the job I wanted, and I was ready for a new challenge.

With help from my parents, we found an apartment, paid for the summer course and registered me with the Accessibility Office. Another example of them being my scaffold! I started the course in May, and my mom came with me to ease the transition on my first day as I met a few of my professors and some of my classmates. Our first day wasn't what I expected. Because it was a television and radio journalism course, we spent our first day at CTV watching a taping of the talk show *The Social*. It was fascinating to see how a live TV show is produced.

I was looking forward to the next chapter of my life where I had the opportunity to face two new challenges: living in a big city by myself and learning about the world of television news. The son of sportscaster Dave Hodge was one of my classmates, and he told me his dad enjoyed the phone interview with me for Spartan Youth Radio back in high school. I had never met Dave Hodge in person, but meeting his son was really cool.

The program was four months rather than two years, so there was a lot of information to take in. Learning how to use the video editing software was tough, and I was given the option to do some audio projects, but I felt the need to try something new. I wanted to improve my camera operating skills because having multiple skills is valuable in the industry.

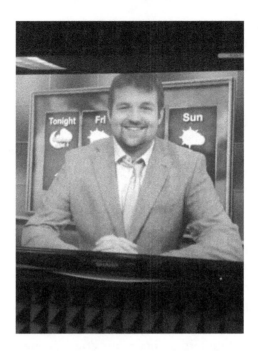

A face for radio (note my tie!)

One of my favourite parts of this course was simulating a live news cast in a television studio at the school. We took turns as anchor, weather reporter, control person and sports reporter, and we would cover whatever news was making headlines that day.

In general, my days in this course went well, but one day was terrible. I had locked myself out of my apartment, and I was really embarrassed. I was unable to concentrate most of the day because I was in the big city without anyone living close by. Because of the anxiety I was facing, I had to take time out from class. My classmates checked on me from time to time, and it felt good to have people look out for me, but I felt like a burden and an inconvenience. One of my classmates wrote: "College and jobs, especially in broadcast journalism, can be fast-paced, high pressure and stressful. Sometimes it's helpful to have a friend to talk to or who will listen when you're feeling stressed. I was a listening ear for Blake sometimes when life was stressful."

Fortunately, one of my professors assured me I wasn't a burden and that I could stay at her place that night if needed. Talk about compassionate. As always, Mom was calm and suggested I stay in a hotel for the night and she would reimburse me, which was a good idea.

Being in distress is nothing to be ashamed of. I thought of what Theresa taught me about how to handle my emotions:

- Practising the breathing techniques for reducing stress always seemed to help. Once settled, going back to recap what happened and using visual metaphors to parallel the learning also helped put in perspective what was once an emotional situation. Sometimes taking those mental images and putting them on paper for future reinforcing seemed to be helpful too.
- Awareness of what we predominantly think and how to manage our emotions is the beginning point to controlling the outcome of our days.
- Mastering breathing techniques directly influences managing emotions and therefore lowering stress in the body.

Eventually my landlord unlocked my door, and my cousin Nick and I got some spare keys cut that night. I also put a sign on the back of my door that said, "Don't forget the keys."

I had been to Toronto multiple times, but I had never lived in a big city before. Even if I had a car, I wouldn't have felt comfortable driving in the city. I didn't need to worry about taking public transit to the grocery store since it was only a few blocks away. I ate most of my meals at the food court at school and other restaurants in the area because there was so much to choose from. On weekends I would often either go to the mall or the movies by myself.

Early in the summer, I went home for a weekend to shoot two public service announcements (PSAs) for the CTV station in Sudbury. The PSAs were about how Espanola has become a friendly and accepting place for those on the autism spectrum, a project that Dennis Lendrum initiated. Making the PSAs gave me a small taste of how a local TV commercial is made. It was fun, but it was a lot of hard work with many retakes after messing up! These PSAs were good additions to my demo reel and my YouTube channel.

The graduation wasn't a big ceremony like at Loyalist. It took place in a small presentation room with guests of our class of eighteen. Dave

Hodge was there, and I got to finally meet him in person. All my professors said they were proud of my accomplishments and the things I had overcome in the course.

It is time now, to pass the mic to one of my Seneca peers, Dr. Joelene Huber, who shared her perspective on having me as a fellow classmate. She also happens to know a thing or two about autism since she's a staff pediatrician at The Hospital for Sick Children and an assistant professor in the faculty of medicine at the University of Toronto:

> I first met Blake when we were both students in the same broadcast journalism program. As a developmental pediatrician, I work with individuals with ASD every day. I diagnose ASD in very young children and follow children throughout childhood and adolescence to monitor their developmental and school progress, ensure resources and supports are in place and advocate for them.
>
> Blake wasn't afraid to say what he thought, which is a really great quality. He shared with me that he had been given a diagnosis of ASD and that when he was young he exhibited echolalia. I was so impressed that he had trouble communicating as a child and now he was in a communications career. Blake also has a great voice for radio.
>
> Knowing Blake's successes, along with the successes of many other adult individuals with ASD, has helped me answer questions when parents of a newly-diagnosed child ask about adult life for individuals with ASD (i.e., when parents ask if their child could ever go to university or college). Some of the early signs associated with a diagnosis of ASD are communication and social skills difficulties. The fact that Blake went to college to pursue a career that is communication-focussed was so

inspiring. I counsel teens with ASD and their parents never to limit themselves, but to do what they love.

The Job Search Continues

With another set of skills to add to my resume and another certificate to hang on my wall, I entered the media battle looking for a full-time job. I continued to see Theresa almost every day for life coaching, and we worked on cover letters, resumes and job applications. I developed a professional demo website at Seneca which had samples of my television reporting and radio talk breaks. I also had a new professional headshot taken. Theresa and I expanded on my effort at getting my professional portfolio out, filling out applications for jobs, making cold calls and setting up informational interviews.

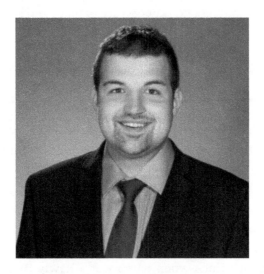

My professional headshot (tie is loose)

I set up an informational interview at the CTV station in northern Ontario. I had been to the studio before so I sort of knew what to expect. I wore my suit and tie (Theresa helped me tie the tie! And it wasn't on for too long!) and met with the news director. There weren't any openings available at the time but meeting the news director was a great way to network and become known in the industry.

During my job search I discovered that Laurentian University had a radio station (CKLU) with a community format where people could host volunteer shows. I quickly pursued the opportunity to host a morning show for the station. I pitched an idea for a show called "Laurentian Mornings" that would play a variety of music and give students updates on local events and news in Sudbury. I was invited in for a tour after which I was excited to start my volunteer show and get some much needed on-air and hosting experience.

During my tenure at CKLU, I continued to look for full-time employment. I found an ad for a freelance journalist for a Sudbury based magazine called *Talent North* which showcases local talent. I sent my portfolio right away so I could make some pocket money and add another item to my resume and portfolio. I immediately knew I was going to enjoy writing for *Talent North*, and showcasing new talent was a lot of fun. The first article I wrote was about the Espanola Little Theatre (ELT) and their successful productions. I had Sharon Sproule to thank for giving me much needed information about the history of ELT and its upcoming performances. I wrote at least ten articles over the course of a few months, and the magazine owner was really impressed with my work.

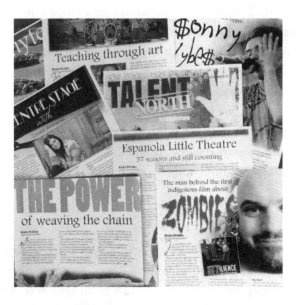

Montage of articles I wrote for *Talent North* **magazine**

Writing articles for *Talent North* and hosting the volunteer CKLU show was fun and I was enjoying myself, but I was still frustrated that no matter what I did, I never got an interview for any jobs I applied for. Once again, I questioned whether my autism was preventing me from getting a media job. I also faced the issue that workplaces often fail to make accommodations for workers on the spectrum or they don't take the time to learn about autism and what employees need. I had been told many times that radio and television are competitive markets that are difficult to get into and I wasn't the only one struggling to get hired. Most of my classmates in both the radio broadcasting and journalism courses were struggling to get work. I felt so fortunate that my parents and Theresa were still there to support me.

I remembered advice that a worker at a radio station in Barrie gave me during an informational interview: if I wanted to get a career in radio, I should take any job that is available. I decided to apply for anything and everything. What did I have to lose? In the meantime, I busied myself with the autism community and was pleased to give a presentation to parents, autistic individuals and service providers on Manitoulin Island.

Another exciting opportunity arose in January of 2016 when we learned that Dr. Temple Grandin would be giving a presentation on autism as well as speaking to farmers about how to handle livestock in a humane way. Dennis Lendrum helped me arrange an interview with Temple before her presentation in Sault Ste. Marie. I was ready to go with some interview questions, I had my digital recorder, and I planned to turn it into a podcast interview for my YouTube Channel and demo website. Meeting Temple Grandin was a huge honour, and I told her so when I started the interview. As you know from the Introduction to this book, we talked about autism and employment.

The Phone Rang!

After two years of sending out resumes, putting together portfolios and demo sites, and doing informational interviews, I finally received the call I had been hoping for. The CEO of a radio station in Yellowknife, Northwest Territories, called to set up an interview with me for a news reporting and host job. I didn't care that it was over three thousand kilometres away because I was desperate for a job, and I was thrilled when I was hired.

Since the station was dedicated to communicating with Indigenous peoples, I needed to learn more about their history and the hardships faced as a result of colonization. Before flying to Yellowknife, my mom arranged for me to meet an elder at Laurentian University to teach me how to show respect when interacting with Indigenous elders when I interviewed them. This was very helpful. I did everything I could to prepare for the next chapter in my life, but would all these preparations help me with my first full-time job? That's what I was about to find out.

North of 60: First Full-Time Career Job

"Facing your toughest challenges and not fearing failure will lead to success."

Me

☆

Although I prepared as much as I could, I had no idea how much this next chapter would shape me into a wiser person.

Dad booked the three flights it took to get to Yellowknife. It was freezing when we arrived—just what I expected in a subarctic climate. It wasn't uncomfortable since I was used to the cold, and I was looking forward to finally experiencing the cool summers up north. I was as nervous for this job as I was excited.

Employers will sometimes meet new workers ahead of time for coffee to get to know them before the first day on the job. Not this time. On the first day I walked into the radio station with another new worker that had been accepted for a similar position. I didn't know anyone or where to start. The supervisor met us and gave an overview of Northwest Territories Indigenous peoples. I expected to be trained on how to cover the news and where to find news stories for the radio station, but I was left to fend for myself. There appeared to be little orientation. It seemed like they expected me to know everything right off the bat. The staff seemed nice, but we didn't have much conversation and everyone kept to themselves.

Dad stayed with me until I moved into my new home, a single bedroom in a house with a shared kitchen and bathroom. My parents had lined up the rental and covered the cost. It was one of the cheapest options available since rent and the overall cost of living is really expensive in the north. My landlords and roommate were nice.

I didn't initially reveal that I was on the spectrum, and when I finally did, my work colleagues didn't think much of it. For the first month or so, things went along pretty well at the station and I got to know the morning show host, Ashley Anthony. Since my ultimate goal was to become a host rather than work in news all the time, she encouraged me to talk to the CEO. Ashley turned out to be the only real friend I made at the station and the person who helped me in my times of need. We are still really good friends. She also complimented me on the stories that I wrote. After a couple of months, I started co-hosting alongside Ashley occasionally, and it soon became daily.

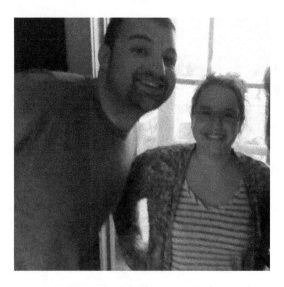

Ashley and me at the station

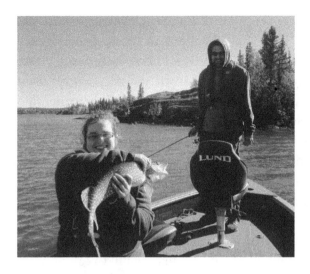

Fishing with Ashley, Great Slave Lake, NWT

Independent but Supported

Co-hosting was no easy feat. I insisted that I announce the weather and current temperatures of communities across the territory but a lot of the names were difficult to pronounce (for example, Tsiigehtchic is pronounced *tsih-gay-chik* and means Arctic Red River) and Ashley would correct me. Writing news stories without a wire service was difficult because we had to write them in our own words. I made a few mistakes with misleading information, which was embarrassing. Ashley wasn't pleased, rightly so. She meant well, but it didn't feel good when she told me I messed up. I would get upset with her at times and throw her criticism in her face because I let my ego take over. But once I calmed down, I said I was sorry, and she accepted my apology. Without Ashley's straightforward constructive criticism, I might not have learned to accept feedback correctly and sharpen my interviewing and research skills, which I needed to do to become the journalist and radio host I am today.

A Tense Workplace

The radio station seemed like the perfect job at first. Everyone was so laid-back and had a good sense of humour, but it soon became clear that there was a lot of unease. Unbeknownst to me, the station had recently been shut down due to funding shortages. There was a lot of tension and ego as well as a history of continued staff turnover. Everyone stuck to their own work and no one ever wanted to work together. I started to notice this about two or three months into the job, but even before then my anxiety and stress levels were a lot higher than they should have been. I started worrying over little things, and some things that didn't bother me for a while started to bother me once again. I started cleaning my desk with alcohol wipes after someone mentioned they had stomach flu. This was the first time in a long time that my OCD fear of germs and getting sick came back. I was also constantly afraid of being fired and losing this job. It got so bad one day that I had to excuse myself to take an anxiety pill to calm myself down. Co-hosting the morning show with Ashley was the best part of this job, but once the morning show was over at 8:00 a.m., my mood changed and I dreaded the idea of another workday.

My biggest problem was not getting along well with one reporter. When we first met, this person was nice. However, after I made the mistake of inadvertently crossing them when I pointed out mistakes in this person's story in a calm positive way, we got into a verbal argument which led to me having a horrific panic attack. I have never handled verbal conflict very well—it's one of my main anxiety triggers. I was afraid I was going to be fired. For the first time in almost a year a panic attack crushed me. I was unable to talk in full sentences and was struggling to breathe. Ashley and another staff member said everything would be okay and that I wasn't going to lose my job over what happened.

Another challenge I had to face was the expectations of the company. In hindsight, I see that they wanted me to hit the ground running and expected me to have more knowledge and experience than I had. I had expected more guidance and orientation. Not a good fit. They wanted me to cover stories outside Yellowknife from all the fly-in communities in the territory, but I wasn't provided with contacts, leads or a travel budget. Developing local contacts would take time, but the expectation was to deliver daily stories.

You don't need to know all the details, but sufficed to say it was a toxic environment for me. I dreaded going to work in the morning, and

I cried myself to sleep some nights and woke up in the morning hating my life. I knew it wasn't all on me because there was continued turnover at the company. My parents said this was all part of the workplace, but it was really difficult to talk to them about how toxic the environment was and how badly I wanted to get out. Sometimes Mom and Dad would be firm and give me the tough love pushes I needed to carry on, but this time Dad could see how depressed and upset I was, so he flew to Yellowknife to visit for a while. We had a great time, but I knew I had to face the music again without his support as soon as he went home.

Bonus—Living in a "Cool" Part of Canada

Living in Yellowknife allowed me to experience a whole new region of Canada. Since I enjoy travelling and seeing new places, this was like killing two birds with one stone. Yellowknife is in the subarctic, which means the sun is almost always up in the summer. Some weekend days I would wake up thinking it was lunchtime only to look at my phone to find out it was three o'clock in the morning. Summer doesn't last long in NWT, only a month or so. The best way to cool off was to go swimming in Great Slave Lake, which was surprisingly warm during the summer, warmer than Lake Superior. Family friends Rachel, Lanny and Grace came from Ontario for a visit, which helped reduce my loneliness. Fishing with Ashley and her family was another great escape from the work stress.

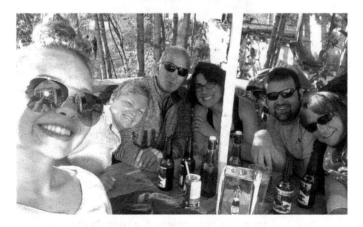

Best family friends and my parents visiting me in Yellowknife

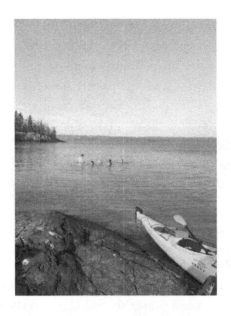

Midnight sun, kayaking and swimming, Great Slave Lake, NWT

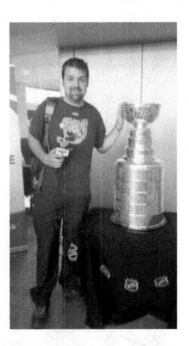

Special treat to interview former NHLers
and touch the Stanley Cup

Positives of the Job

I covered some newsworthy stories. Besides the Stanley Cup and former NHL stars coming to Yellowknife, and interviewing Adam Growe of Cash Cab fame, I featured a local disability awareness event hosted by the NWT Disabilities Council at their 38th Annual Benefit Auction. Another highlight was learning about Indigenous peoples' lives in NWT from the language elders at the station.

On the day of my six-month review, my boss told me that my co-hosting was good but I had shortcomings and needed to report original local and NWT-wide stories rather than writing my own version of stories I found online. Ashley appreciated my stories since she often had to rush on her own to find stories for the morning news. I was upset, but I was thankful they extended my probation another three months. Because my goal was to find and report on my own stories, I decided to focus on making contacts in Yellowknife and the surrounding communities. Thinking outside the box, I developed my own business cards and walked throughout town distributing my cards and introducing myself. I also introduced myself virtually in other towns and communities throughout NWT.

A few weeks before Christmas as I waited anxiously to see if I would pass my probation extension and stay on permanently, I got a call one Sunday night from the station technician. He wanted to know if I was ready for our trip to Fort Resolution, leaving early the next morning, to repair the transmitter. I was caught off guard. I didn't know anything about the trip. My boss had said nothing about it, and I hadn't checked my work phone over the weekend since I had never been texted before on the weekend. Normally when it comes to going on a business trip in most workplaces, a boss or supervisor that organizes the trip meets with the employee ahead of time so that plans can be made. I was unprepared, but I packed an overnight bag and some snacks for the trip. We left before dawn and drove five hours. On the way we came across many wood bison herds and a small herd of woodland caribou—exciting!

The next day I went around town to hand out my contact information so that if people had local news they wanted covered they could contact me. Students from the local school had fun creating liners for me to introduce them on the station.

When we got back from the work road trip my agonizing wait was over. After a long day at work, I would finally learn my fate. It was a killer right from the start. I had butterflies in my tummy and hadn't slept well the previous few nights. I felt like I had done what I could by covering stories and getting my contact information out to people. While my immediate supervisor had emailed me and recommended that I be hired permanently, the final decision lay with the boss—who had a different response. I was let go because they needed someone who could work more independently and had more experience.

Initially, I assumed I was let go because of my autism, but they reiterated that I didn't have what they were looking for. I was relieved but devastated, and I held back tears for the remainder of the meeting. I wanted to get angry and yell and insult, but I didn't. I pulled myself together, took a deep breath and thanked them for giving me such an amazing opportunity. I shook their hands and left the office.

The walk home was only a few blocks, but it felt longer. I didn't know what I was going to tell my parents, and I felt like I had embarrassed not only myself but my entire family. Had I messed up my life for good? I was under the impression that if someone was fired from a job the chances of landing another one are unlikely. Deep down I knew that wasn't true because many people have found new jobs and become successful after a setback, but it was my first time so I was rightfully concerned about my future.

Everything was so uncertain. Would I ever work in media again? Would I have to work a menial job the rest of my life? Was I a failure? In a way I was happy that I didn't have to work there anymore because it really was a toxic environment, but it was disappointing to leave this way. I told my parents the news over the phone. I was so worried about what they would say, but they were proud of me for everything that I did, and they assured me that my career in media wasn't over but just beginning.

I was deeply saddened and disturbed with everything that had transpired, and I had more drinks than I should have that night. I ended up calling a local crisis phone line because for the first time in a long time I was having thoughts of suicide. I really didn't want to kill myself, but I was in a lot of pain and needed to talk to someone professional to get help. I wanted to live, but I also wanted to get rid of the pain. I explained my situation to the person on the other end of the line, and she did a wonderful job keeping me calm and making me feel better. When I ended the conversation, it occurred to me that in the movie *Cast Away*, Chuck Noland wanted to end it all because he felt he would never get off the island he was stranded on, but one day the tide came in and gave him a piece of plastic that he used as a makeshift sail to get off the island. He said, "You have to keep breathing because tomorrow the sun will rise. Who knows what the tide could bring?"

Dad arrived a few days later to offer me emotional support and help pack my things. The station offered to keep me on until the end of January, but I decided to move on. Ashley explained the full situation to Dad to give him a better idea of what had happened over the past ten months, which made things clearer. Dad was very pleased that I continued to go to work despite all the stuff I had been through. I am so thankful that my father came all the way to Yellowknife to help me during this difficult time.

On my last day at the station, I hosted the morning show with Ashley one last time. After work, Ashley and I grabbed a bite to eat at a nearby café, and I ordered a mug of hot chocolate that had whipped cream on top with a heart drawn on it with chocolate. I took a picture of it and posted it to Facebook saying, "Even in dark times, kindness will always prevail."

Ashley is a great friend who helped me in my time of need and accepted me for who I am. We are still friends and keep in touch.

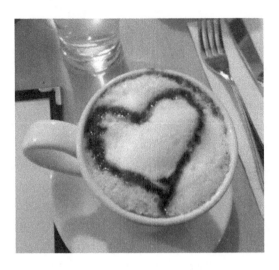

Always look for the good

Losing my first job in Yellowknife didn't ruin my life. I did what many autistic people would likely not do and tried something outside my comfort zone. I tried new things. I saw new places. If it weren't for this experience, which was ultimately a stepping-stone for my career, I may still be living in Mom and Dad's basement. Sure, things were still uncertain and I didn't know what would happen next, but I would continue to learn, grow and gain experience.

I am going to hand the mic over to Ashley, Mom and Dad who shared their points of view of this chapter of my life.

Ashley:

> At first Blake was timid and shy, but then he started to find his voice. It was a difficult atmosphere to navigate with a lot of hostility and ego, but he tried to blend in.

> Blake was very stuck in his ways. He always had to have things a particular way, and he would ask a lot of questions for clarification. I remember one morning on our way to work the sun was rising and I stopped at the Bush Pilot's Monument. Blake was confused because it was not the normal place and because I had burst out

of the car to run up this huge set of stairs to the top of the monument. Blake followed behind so timidly, but once we got to the top, we spent a few minutes there enjoying the beauty of the north and Great Slave Lake.

I think the most difficult thing I have encountered so far in my adult life is when Blake was being bullied. I remember sitting on the front porch of the station talking with another person, and there was an eruption from inside. Blake walked out stark white in the face and had a breakdown. By this time, we were already good friends and it was tough to see him like that.

There were a lot of instances where Blake would misinterpret or miscommunicate what people were trying to say. Some people would not take the time to understand what he was saying or to explain what is going on. I think the best approach to helping Blake cope was to treat him with the respect that any person deserves, as well as patiently explain what was going on in a way he could understand.

What I would say to future employers and work colleagues of Blake's is: don't be an ignorant asshole. Lol—it's the best way to put it. Take some time, ask questions, learn to do things a different way to help the autistic person with transitions and new information.

When I found out Blake was autistic it changed my view of him and other people on the spectrum. I knew little about autism and what came along with it. Blake has proven to be an outstanding friend, an amazing person and a fantastic co-host. When Blake taught me about autism, I gained so much respect for him and his perseverance to help other people understand.

Blake is a super tough individual with a lot of drive and compassion, and I am really proud of him for going through all of that crap and coming out with his head held high. Most people couldn't muster half of the integrity he has.

Ashley left the station a few months after I did. On to greener pastures for both of us!

Mom:

In some ways we may have contributed to Blake's failure at this job. How? Two ways. First, by inadvertently setting him up to believe that his employer would provide him with solid on-boarding, training and orientation. Ted and I came from large employers that had extensive orientation for new hires, especially recent graduates. At my workplace, orientation training took weeks and weeks with mentors to go to after the new employee got their feet wet on tasks.

Secondly, I think the whole issue of disclosure is full of pitfalls for the new employee/interviewee and the employer. When one has an invisible disability like ASD, if you disclose during your interview chances are the phone won't ring for a callback. If you are fortunate enough to get hired, when do you inform about your disability? After your probation? What if you need a few simple accommodations to make you succeed but don't want to ask for them in case you are being singled out?

This time in Yellowknife taught Blake:

- There are always going to be assholes at work. The key is to learn not to be one and to stay away from them!
- To learn to control one's anger.

- To handle feedback more constructively.
- To ask for help—it's a sign of strength, not weakness.
- To disclose his autism alongside strategies to succeed.

Dad:

What Blake experienced was a bunch of life lessons that have made him stronger. It was painful to witness from afar. Since I'm usually a guy who doesn't spend a lot of time talking through issues, every week or two I would send a wise quote to help him through this challenging work experience. Below are some of the sayings I sent Blake to give him some comfort in knowing he wasn't alone. After all, "What doesn't kill us, makes us stronger."

- Stop being afraid of what could go wrong and start being excited about what could go right.
- Difficult roads often lead to beautiful destinations.
- Criticism may not be agreeable, but it is necessary. It fulfills the same function as pain in the human body, it calls attention to an unhealthy state of things.
- Tough times don't last, tough people do.

North of 53: Arctic Radio and The Pas

The year ended on a high note with a wonderful Christmas and New Years celebrated with my family. It was time to get my life back in order and start the next chapter. Everything was uncertain for me once again, just like it was when I started to look for my first job. It seemed like I was back to square one. In hindsight, I was back at the beginning but with more workplace and radio industry experience.

I wasn't going to get my next radio job sitting around doing nothing. I set up countless phone interviews and resumed freelancing for *Talent North*. That was a lot of fun, and I got to meet new people. One of my favourite interviews was with sci-fi author Brian Horeck. I also wrote an article featuring Jenna Carter, an artist who painted a picture of my grandparent's cottage which I gave them for Christmas.

In March 2017, I interviewed for a job at a radio station in The Pas, northern Manitoba, to work as a news reporter. Even though it wasn't a hosting job, I felt the need to think "outside the box" and apply with hopes that I could get a hosting opportunity while working in the news. They offered me the job and said I could also host a show or do some voiceover work on a volunteer basis. This made me want to accept the job right away, but I wasn't sure how good I would be at covering the news because I had needed help at my previous job with getting information accurate. My confidence had been crushed. I felt I was better at covering human interest stories. I was upfront with the employer that I would benefit from solid mentoring and that I was eager to learn and receive advice to be a better news reporter and announcer. Mom and Dad assured me I would do just fine. I accepted the job offer, and before I knew it I was on my way to The Pas.

Mom, Dad and I did a road trip to The Pas, which took about three days from Espanola. We stopped in Thunder Bay and Winnipeg as well. When we arrived, I could see that The Pas was a lot like Espanola, with the small northern town feeling I love. I could tell I was going to enjoy this place. We stayed in a nice hotel for the first few days before moving into an apartment my employer helped find. I would finally have my own space, and the rent was much cheaper than in Yellowknife. My mom said my apartment was so much nicer than her first one, which was in a dingy basement full of cockroaches!

A Family Radio Station Extraordinaire

The day before I officially started work, the assistant manager, Chris, and I had breakfast so I could get to know him. He was so nice and made me feel welcome and somewhat less nervous about my new job and my new home. Overall, Manitoba's people are very welcoming and laid-back and friendly—they don't call it Friendly Manitoba for nothing! Everyone wants to look out for you and make sure you're happy.

The first day of my new job was a lot different than my first day in Yellowknife. They didn't expect me to know everything and hit the ground running without training. Arctic Radio, the company that runs the radio station in The Pas and two other stations in the province (Flin Flon and Thompson), is family run, and they treated me like family from the start. The employees looked out for one another and pitched in to help whenever they could. The outgoing news director for the station started training me immediately and showed me step by step how the news runs at the station and gave me a list of local contacts. He introduced me to the mayor of The Pas on the first day and showed me other useful tricks for covering the news. I am thankful for all the help I received, and I started to feel comfortable almost immediately.

I could go on and on about how positive my experience and my life has been in The Pas. A few highlights at Arctic Radio include having met local MP Niki Ashton, MLA Amanda Lathlin, and Opaskwayak Ininew Christian Sinclair. I covered local stories that will become the history of tomorrow, like the Town Centre Hotel fire, the local minor hockey team winning the Chevrolet Good Deeds Cup, and events at the Northern Manitoba Trappers' Festivals. My work has become noticed locally, and people have commended me for my news coverage. I have learned skills and strategies that are helping me to be successful and accurate in my reporting. For example, I call certain news sources and review the stories I plan to put on the air. It pays off because local politicians respect me for caring about the quality of the stories. At a special event in town, the local dignitaries invited me to sit at their table, an honour that means I am doing pretty damn good in this industry after all.

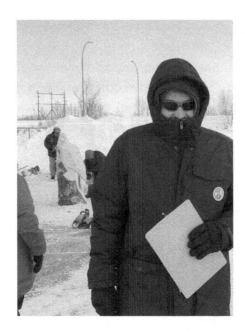

On remote location, -30°C, at chainsaw carving event, Northern Manitoba Trappers' Festival, The Pas, MB

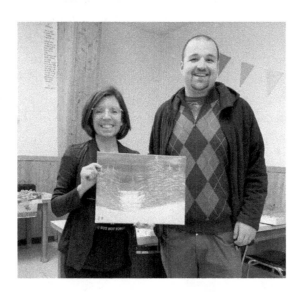

MP Niki Ashton receiving one of my landscape paintings

At our radio station everyone tries to pitch in whenever they can even if it means working outside their position. Colleagues offer me stories almost everyday, and even though I don't always use them, it's great that we work as a team. In return, I help them with ideas for sales or contests or with commercial voicing and production. I am also available to fill in and do voice tracking if someone is sick. They really appreciate it when I help out and show initiative without being asked.

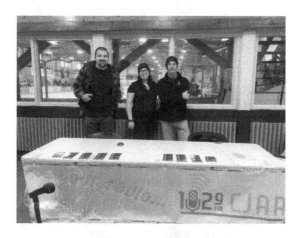

On location at Opaskwayak Cree Nation (OCN) Jr A hockey game *(courtesy Arctic Radio)*

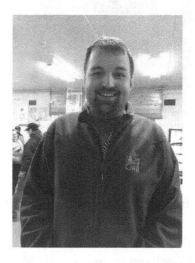

Out in the community

Not only does this company treat people like family, but they are also more than happy to help their employees solve and overcome problems to ensure we do our jobs better. My employer provided me with a checklist to follow before sending the news each day to make sure that the spelling and numbers are accurate. I often use this helpful resource while proofreading stories.

Like in most workplaces I have been given constructive criticism and positive feedback to make me a better news reporter and radio personality. This includes remembering how to talk with a conversational voice on air and adding voice clips to news stories. The best bit of feedback I received was when my employer said the news is the best it's been in a long time since I started working there. These kind words made me feel proud and successful. When anyone makes a mistake on air we simply apologize and fix it or just laugh if it is harmless!

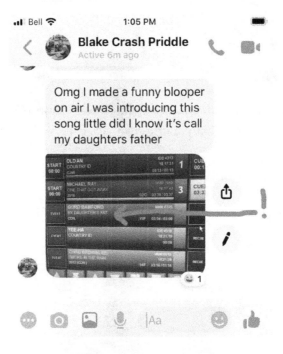

Gord Bamford's daughter is not fat LOL

The company also organizes dinners when someone leaves the company, as well as pool and casino nights. We have had Christmas parties with lots of yummy food, good drinks, fun games like Cards Against Humanity and secret Santa gift exchanges. The station makes a real effort to ensure we all feel valued.

You may be wondering about whether I have told my employer I am autistic…Yes, I disclosed my autism and the challenges I have. I also told them what works for me to do a good job. Our *Morning Wake Up* host even interviewed me to promote World Autism Awareness Day. After all, awareness leads to understanding and inclusion close to home.

A Great Community Too

The Pas is a small town just like the one I grew up in. There is the occasional jackass out there (and everywhere!), but most people care for each other and are friendly. One time when my parents and I were eating supper outside a local chip stand, a worker gave our dog a bowl of water, which was very thoughtful. My Gramps says that folks in the *real* north are straightforward, hardy and have a strong sense of community; we can't rely on anyone but ourselves since we live so far away from cities.

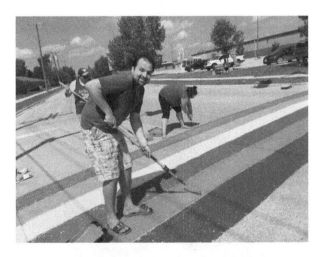

Helping where I can

You might be surprised, but what I dislike about living in the *real* north is that the winters are longer and colder than in northern Ontario, so it can be difficult to enjoy winter activities because of the biting wind chill. By March, the weather is warmer and there are lots of ice fishing derbies. I have been in two of them and had fun even though I only caught one fish. Gramps flew up one weekend to fish just as the ice left the lake—in June!

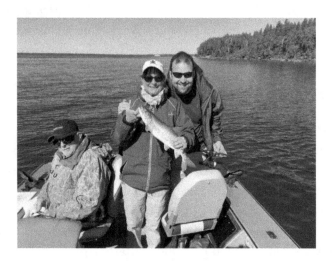

Fishing with Gramps, Mom, me on Clearwater Lake, MB

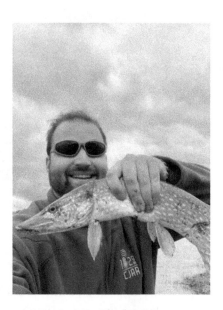

My first fish, North Saskatchewan River

Thankfully, there are lots of indoor activities in The Pas for us to stay warm. Playing darts at the local Legion is a highlight, as is bingo. I have played pool at the local pool hall, and the owner of the pool hall even took the time to teach me how to hold a pool cue properly and how to make a good shot. The local junior hockey teams also provide some indoor entertainment, and they always put on a good show (and the arena has good food to eat). While it's a flight away for both of us, my dad has even met me in Winnipeg for a weekend where we took in a CFL Bombers' game.

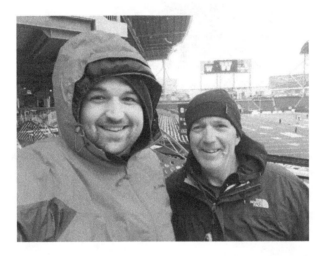

A weekend with Dad in Winnipeg cheering on the Bombers

Manitoba is known for its mosquitoes! They are in abundance in our area especially during the late spring and summer months, which prevents many people from going into the bush. But when they are gone by early fall, there are lots of great places to hunt, which I do most weekends. I've even bagged a few partridge. I met a great guy who works with Ducks Unlimited, and he has taken me goose hunting, which is fun. I got two on my first day. We have scouted an area for deer hunting, too, and I'm still holding out for a Manitoba buck.

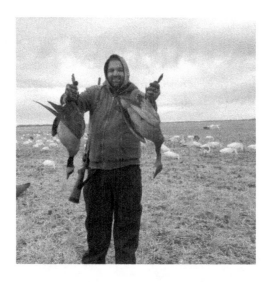

First successful goose hunt, MB

The cost of living here is reasonable, and I can afford car insurance for my new *used* car. Having a car is useful because it is easier to bring home shopping and I can take a drive anytime I want without calling a cab or asking for a ride. I surprised my parents by getting the car serviced and winter tires installed when it was due without being prompted.

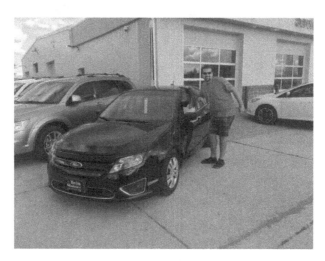

My first new *used* car!

I really enjoy my job at Arctic Radio and living in The Pas. I continue to gain valuable experience at work and in life. I am a lot happier with my life now, and I really look forward to what will come next!

Living Alone through COVID-19

"No one should ever say 'My life is ruined' when something bad happens. If you're still alive and still breathing, your life is far from ruined. There will always be a rainbow at the end of the storm."

Me

☆

After working in The Pas, Manitoba, for four years, I gained the experience needed to cover the biggest news events of the century—the COVID-19 pandemic. Working in a small-town radio station often means updating the news maybe once per day, but during the pandemic I had to update the news several times daily and work hard to keep people informed.

I had a small taste of what Walter Cronkite had to go through when JFK was assassinated and what the news reporters on 9/11 had to go through updating the news while maintaining composure. Just when I thought I could catch a break, new information would come up on the wires. When JFK was killed the coverage slowed after three days, but this pandemic has dominated the news for a long time and seems endless. I have become overwhelmed and anxious and have lost the energy to do things I enjoy. I had to take a break from hosting volunteer shows to focus on the news and recharge my batteries whenever I could.

One day was so overwhelming I had to take some deep breaths before I had a panic attack. I managed to pull myself together, and I gave as much coverage as I could to the listeners, but I knew that my troubles would start again very soon. I was worried about what would happen to my parents and family, when I would see them again and if

I would become sick. My fear of germs isn't as bad as it used to be, but anything can happen. Talking to my boss Chris, and Mom and Dad about my issues has helped me feel better. And I know that a therapist is just a phone call away if I need to talk.

I have had to deal with people who are paranoid and stressed from the pandemic. Many people have said they felt like they were in a sci-fi movie or it's the worst thing that's ever happened in the world. It may be the worst thing my generation has lived through, but I'm sure earlier generations and recent immigrants from war-torn countries have had it harder. People were forced to fight and shoot people in World War II, and many died. During the London Blitz people had to build bomb shelters in their backyards or hide in tube stations hoping they would survive another day. During 9/11 people were trapped alive in the World Trade Center rubble thinking they were going to die. I thought about these events to help me put my COVID-19 experience into perspective.

During the COVID-19 pandemic many have had it tough worrying about jobs, illness and dying. Most of us were just told to stay home and watch TV, paint a picture, play the guitar or even go out into the wilderness to do outdoor activities while physical distancing. I really haven't had it that hard. I spend most weekends at home recharging my batteries regardless of what is happening in the world.

Overall, I helped people stay informed during the pandemic, made a difference and contributed to society during such a difficult time. Dad told me not to look at this crisis as a sprint, but more like a marathon.

The pandemic is still going on as I write this, but it has shown us what really matters in life. It has taught us valuable lessons and given us wake-up calls which would have only been possible with a pandemic. Nature started to make a recovery. Families started to realize what it's like to be a family. For too long, adults went to work and kids went to school with little quality time together. Kids learned at home and adults who have been able to, worked from home. We are also learning where the cracks are in our society, and what we need our governments to focus on to protect everyone post-pandemic.

I also hope the pandemic will make people realize that even though we are not living in the Middle Ages and we have better health care, it doesn't mean we are invincible. The next time we come across an unknown virus, I hope we'll apply the lessons we are learning from COVID-19 and enact new measures to prevent a similar crisis.

My attitude toward life comes partially from my Grandma Dot, who, when faced with hardship, always said, "This too shall pass." So, the next time we face a tragedy, if we keep breathing and stick together, we can make it through anything as long as we have the will to live.

My mom's journal entry below reflects what is likely a worry all parents can relate to:

What a resilient kid we have!

Week five of the pandemic shutdown, and it's Tuesday morning after Easter. I start my daily routine—turn on CJAR to listen to the morning show followed by the news at noon by Blake Priddle. It's a lovely way to hear your kid's voice every day when he reads the news from 2300 km away. Ted and I also joke to ourselves: "Oh good, he got to work today!"

This morning the host said that Blake Priddle is away today. *What?* Blake is never away from work. Panic sets in. I text, call, messenger—no answer. Give it thirty minutes; can't wait any longer. I PM the host (I know it appears I am a helicopter Mom who should back off and NOT ever call a kid's work colleague, but these are different times and Blake is a different kid, I reason). Within seconds the host responds (*thank you!*).

"Yeah, Blake came in first thing this morning but wasn't feeling well, so left. I'm sure he's okay."

My heart rate slows and my palms stop sweating. I text Ted this good, albeit second-hand update.

Three hours later, I get a text from Blake apologizing for not responding. He says he's full of chills, aches, headache, nausea. It started Monday.

"Do you have any Tylenol? Soup? Crackers? Ginger ale? Clean sheets? Tissue?" I ask.

Worried Mom from SO FAR AWAY.

Tuesday turns to Wednesday, into Thursday, into Friday. Still sick.

I am a bad mom—I missed sixteen calls (damn silent feature inadvertently on). Instant angst, bile creeps up my throat.

Blake gets a hold of Ted who talks him off his anxiety-laden ledge.

"No, Blake, you can't get fired for missing work because you are sick…No, Blake, your mom and I are healthy and practising physical distancing and handwashing."

Five days with a fever. The government self-assessment tool prompts Blake to get a COVID-19 test. Lots of chats ensue to reassure him while he waits for results. And he waits.

Thankfully, Blake begins to feel better—not 100%, but better.

Northern communities are at heightened risk. Co-morbidities exist in higher rates than southern urban neighbours in the form of inequities—poverty, intergenerational Indigenous trauma from colonization and lack of services. The closest ICU is an eight-hour drive to Winnipeg. In an effort to stop the transmission of COVID-19, the Manitoba government bans all non-essential travel "north of 53," so we couldn't drive to take care of Blake if we wanted to.

Blake's boss, Chris (*Thanks Chris!*), drops off soup and ginger ale. Blake's first interaction in over a week. Talk about a caring workplace!

Six days after the COVID-19 test, it comes back negative. Back to work he goes after being off two weeks.

Fast forward six months, August 2020, and Blake's anxiety is kicking in. He misses a few days of work—likely due to worrying himself sick. He's worrying from afar because his parents are on a road trip to visit his isolated grandpa.

Fast forward a year into the pandemic, and Blake is going on two years between vacations. Travel bans and lockdowns—both important since his community has exploded with COVID-19 cases (over nine hundred for a population around 11,500).

The world holds its breath and waits for effective treatments, vaccines and warmer weather.

There's isolation and then there's ISOLATION. We all have to practise physical distancing and wear masks. Blake's OCD and anxiety disorder (germs are a trigger and my parents are in danger and I'm gonna lose my job) kick into overdrive. Ted and I, from 2300 km away, do our best to calm and reassure him, all the while not sugar-coating that this pandemic is a real threat and the science is still evolving on what this is really about.

Local community radio stations are a lifeline for many folks in times like these. Announcers and news reporters are deemed essential workers. Blake's station provides up-to-date COVID-19 information daily, in English and Cree. The northern Manitoba family-owned Arctic Radio set of three stations are to be commended for staying the course despite (I'm sure) dwindling ad revenue, the lifeblood of commercial stations.

When we scroll through social media sites there are many tips to keep our mental well-being in check during these unprecedented times. One tip that keeps surfacing is to limit oneself to COVID-19 news for one time throughout the day. In other words, don't have CBC News or CNN on all day. This will help keep anxiety, grief, depression at bay, the experts say.

So, what happens if you are the news guy who has to research, write and read these COVID-19 updates fourteen times a day, five days a week over weeks and months? Every night you go home to your apartment, live alone and isolate? How would you do with OCD, anxiety and being autistic with no family within a three-day drive? Blake is the most resilient person Ted and I know. WE ARE BEYOND PROUD.

Since COVID-19 has seeped into everyone's lives around the world, you can't really get away from it. Being on social media every day, I read about many autistic families struggling with services being cut, online schooling with no accommodations and supports, anxiety through the roof and so on. Here's a sample of a chat I had while trying to lend a sympathetic ear:

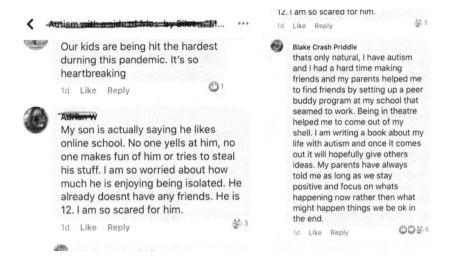

12. I am so scared for him.

Our kids are being hit the hardest durning this pandemic. It's so heartbreaking

1d   Like   Reply

Adrian W
My son is actually saying he likes online school. No one yells at him, no one makes fun of him or tries to steal his stuff. I am so worried about how much he is enjoying being isolated. He already doesnt have any friends. He is 12. I am so scared for him.

1d   Like   Reply

12. I am so scared for him.
1d   Like   Reply

Blake Crash Priddle
thats only natural, I have autism and I had a hard time making friends and my parents helped me to find friends by setting up a peer buddy program at my school that seamed to work. Being in theatre helped me to come out of my shell. I am writing a book about my life with autism and once it comes out it will hopefully give others ideas. My parents have always told me as long as we stay positive and focus on whats happening now rather then what might happen things we be ok in the end.

1d   Like   Reply

Tweets showing how pandemic affects autistics and families

Time for Creativity

One positive outcome many of us have experienced while living through a pandemic is time on our own. With lockdown after lockdown, I put my alone time to good use by painting landscapes and creative writing western-themed short stories. I continued to think about the complex and often competing opinions of the autism community, so I decided to put my ideas on paper on how to bridge the opposing viewpoints by pitching a TV show:

TV Show Pitch: The Missing Piece of Autism

Premise: How can we try to get polarized folks in the autism community to see each other's perspectives in a respectful way?

Genre: Reality and Education

Duration: one hour per episode, four episode/part series.

Outline: There are a lot of self-advocates on the "higher end" of the autism spectrum who are very proud of who they are (rightfully so). Some are especially vocal and are vehemently against any form of treatment or the curing of any autistic traits, however minor or severe. Many ascribe to the neurodiversity movement where being autistic is an identity not to be tinkered with in any way. Society's barriers are the problem to be changed, not the autistic person.

Some folks we will call "severely" autistic may require twenty-four-hour care and be unable to look after themselves. As a result, some parents voice that they want an all-out cure (or a cure from the challenging symptoms).

Both "sides" of this issue are strong in their convictions. Much hatred has spilled into the social media autism community, which is awfully difficult to listen to when you are an autistic person.

Autism is a *spectrum* disorder. The common belief is that once you've met one person with autism, you've met one person with autism, meaning no two people behave the same because they are autistic. Who are we to judge how parents feel about their children? But it could be a slippery slope. The word "cure" conjures up a hot mess of emotions. Does wanting a cure (be it all variants/forms of autism or just a cure for the "harmful" traits) make this an irreconcilable issue?

Format: This limited four-part series is inspired by the TV documentary called *First Contact* which followed various white Canadians who had strong opinions about Indigenous peoples. Over the course of the series their views changed once they learned about white privilege, colonialism and reconciliation. This show will have a similar format. It will follow four to six autistic self-advocating adults who openly have strong views about parents who are looking for an "autism cure" and want their children to change. Self-advocates often see these people as selfish and prejudiced without fully understanding what they go through. The self-advocates will follow the footsteps of caregivers and people with *severe* autism. Similarly, the parents of severely autistic children (from toddler, teen to adult) will spend time with other self-advocates to learn their worldviews. The intent of the series is to bridge the polarizing stands and bring a measure of empathy to both perspectives. The show itself is not advocating for a cure but to educate people who are unaware of the various forms autism can take.

The show would conclude with both groups visiting Channel-Port aux Basques, Newfoundland, the most autism-friendly place in Canada.

A show like this would help open important discussions about the different ways people view autism. I will always have high hopes for people with autism, the same way my parents had for me.

...

Now that I have outlined my life and its successes and challenges in chronological order, my family, friends and I will use the next chapter to share our perspectives on various issues that relate to my journey and no doubt others' journeys too.

Chapter 5:

Define "Normal" & Other Thoughts

What is "Normal" Anyway?

**"Just because you can't see autism doesn't
mean people don't have it."**

Me

☆

My mom has spent over twenty years shining a light on a particular form of discrimination called "ableism," which is a form of discrimination against individuals with disabilities. While society has been calling out most "isms"—racism, sexism, ageism—for some time, ableism is one of the last to be tackled. The disability movement has worked tirelessly to make the world a fair and equitable place. One of the ways to do this is to address the language people use. "Ableist" language assumes disabled people are inferior to nondisabled people. In the case of ASD, ableist words imply autism is bad and needs to be fixed. Describing autism in this way has negative effects on how society views and treats autistic people and may even negatively affect how autistic folks see themselves. Many of us don't even realize we are using ableist words or phrases, and for this reason we need to pay attention to what we say.

> Did you know? The word "normal" is only about 150 years old? It's a socially-constructed term that was used as the fields of psychiatry and psychology began to label those who are different, with and without visible disabilities.

Academics, like my mom, say there is an evolution in how society views the "disabled." In a nutshell, there are at least three models. Many argue that the first two (Medical and Functional) are outdated and need to be replaced by the third model, The Social Model of Disability.

Medical Model	Functional Model	Social Model
Cures/treats the problem/illness	Fixes/changes the person/behaviours	Removes societal barriers to include those with differences

Some people feel individuals who are affected so severely with certain traits and behaviours will never fully participate in society even if all societal barriers were to be removed. They advocate for a cure to the problem or illness and welcome advances in the medical field and knowledge that can lead to improvements. For example, if someone has profound autism, needs round-the-clock supervision, has no sense of danger and is unable to communicate their needs, then making accommodations to the external environment probably would not change their life. But new medical treatments may bring relief to extreme sensory processing difficulties. My mom and I believe there is merit in bits of each of these models and see them as complementary, not either or. ASD is a spectrum, and when we talk about autism, we need to remember the diversity of the spectrum. We need to honour and respect each person's worldview.

Neurodiversity is an interesting term I use and promote, but it is not universally accepted. Neurodiversity views autism as an identity, like sexual orientation, not a developmental disorder or disability. So, it means that we aren't to be fixed, it's our environment that needs fixing.

From Dennis Lendrum, grandparent and autism advocate:

> In 2005, our grandson was diagnosed with autism. I did not even know what the meaning of the word was at that time. I was advised to speak with Jo Beyers as apparently her son Blake has autism. She advised that I should be trying to change the opinions of the political minds. Off we went to Queens Park to meet with MPPs. Within a month, our grandson magically moved way up on the autism services waitlist.

A few years later, I initiated a local group, Autism Acceptance, to draw attention to programs needed in our town. We organized fun family events which included appearances by Crystal Shawanda, government dignitaries, local hockey players, a hockey game, bowling, swimming and lunch. This was the perfect stage for Blake to share his life story as the keynote speaker. I truly hope our grandson can gain the confidence around others that Blake has worked very hard at.

Over the decades my mom has learned and changed her opinions related to autism a lot. Here's what she said:

It is my understanding that the neurodiversity culture promotes that all brains work differently. When Blake was little, I had no idea that stimming and no eye contact were behaviours that shouldn't be corrected. I have learned about the exhaustion that comes with masking/camouflaging what comes naturally, when society forces autistics to fit in by acting "normal." I have learned to be more aware of sensory needs, not force eye contact, that stimming is important, and that it is okay to have the occasional information dump!

Words we use to label and describe the world around us and who inhabits our space is ever-evolving. What is politically correct (PC) today may be wrong in a decade. There has been movement recently to use "first-person language" (i.e., a "person with diabetes" rather than a "diabetic"). My mom started to say, "Blake has autism" rather than, "Blake is autistic." Well, after she checked with me, she course-corrected! I told her, "Mom, I'm autistic! I have no problem being called autistic, that's a part of me." But someone else might feel differently about this.

There is emphasis these days to use strengths-based language as much as possible as opposed to deficits-based words. I can't keep up with all the words I'm supposed to use and not use! For example:

Instead of	Use
Severe	Extensive
Special needs	Needs
Deficit	Challenge
Symptom	Trait
Red flags	Early signs

I refer to myself as "high-functioning," but my mom has sent me articles that recommend not using that term. Society naïvely interprets it to mean verbal and intelligent, which implies those who are non-verbal must be of low intelligence and unable to communicate, and thus "low-functioning." It further implies that the "high-functioning" autistic person has no challenges. Not true! Regardless of what terms we use, it is important to realize that "high-functioning autism" (HFA) is not synonymous with "mild."

Most people with ASD have challenges. Some neurotypicals (NTs) are confused when we show our odd behaviours since we often pass for "normal" in many situations. This causes us stress. While people with more severe autism are not expected to just suck it up and get through difficult moments, HFAs are. I am aware that I have difficulties in a bunch of ways:

- I have trouble understanding verbal instructions (so I need checklists and reminders; instructions broken into smaller bits).
- I have trouble controlling my emotions. I react with rudeness when stressed or confused (and then my OCD kicks in and I apologize a lot).
- Conversations are difficult, especially with more than one person at a time in a noisy place.
  - I often don't understand everything people are really saying.
  - It's difficult to figure out things like sarcasm and facial expressions.
  - It's difficult to make and keep friends.

- The OCD icky intrusive thoughts—many, many times in a day—make it difficult to focus at work. This leaves me tired and not wanting to do stuff. Sometimes they make me depressed.
- I experience small and big panic attacks.

So yeah, I'm high-functioning, but I come with challenges—that can be overcome.

Takeaway lesson: If in doubt, ask the person how they would like to be described!

Me as Teacher—Who Knew?!

Many contributors to this book stated that they have learned a lot about autism, being different, acceptance and inclusion since they met me. The passage of time has allowed some to self-reflect on this. It sounds ironic, but my special education elementary teacher, Robin Spry, said that I taught her!:

A situation that scared me to death in the beginning turned out to be the single most impactful experience of my career. Although my official title was teacher and it was my job to impart knowledge to Blake, in reality, I was the student, the one who learned so much, from him. Blake taught me some of the most valuable life and work lessons. He taught me the importance of empathy for others, the value of perseverance, the meaning of integrity and the joys and headaches that come with standing up for what is right. He taught me humility.

From Blake and his parents, I learned more than five years of university ever taught me. I watched him grow into his own. He worked so hard, tried new things, put himself out there. Blake did what lots of kids can't ever do, and he did it with obstacles to overcome. His grit, resiliency, perseverance and confidence have served him well. He has grown into a fine young man. I am so proud of him, and he should be very proud of himself. Best of all, I made a lifelong friend!

Teaching Blake has been one of the greatest pleasures of my career.

Agreeing to Disagree

The one good thing about increased autism awareness is there is lots of information and opinion. The crummy part is the autism community can be fragmented because of polar opposite opinions on many issues.

My mom and I have been pulled into the social media fray and have learned that just because someone has a differing stand than me doesn't mean we hate them. We can and should simply agree to disagree. While on social media, it is difficult but important to pick one's battles and not get into cyber-bullying with trolls. Many well-intentioned autistic self-advocates oppose any discussion of words like "high-functioning" or "severe" and promote neurodiversity as the umbrella covering all who are autistic. This is where the conflict arises. Parents who feel this doesn't reflect their non-verbal, self-injurious autistic child are often at odds with the other.

My mom stated:

> Personally, I write as a parent because that is who I am. I am not autistic and never for a millisecond would presume to speak on behalf of Blake. But, at the same time, I have thoughts and experiences as a mom raising a child on the spectrum and no one can deny me that. You may disagree, good for you. But you can't deny me reflection on my own experiences. Does what I say or believe hurt others on the spectrum? I don't know. I can't speak for them. If what I write hurts someone, I do apologize, it is not my intent. We may have differing ideas about what is best for those who are "different" (whatever that means), but I know in my heart these

ideas arise out of love and compassion for everyone, wherever one fits on the vast autism spectrum.

My parents and I often have text chats. Here's one my mom and I engaged in late one evening that illustrates this issue:

Me:

I want to give all parents and caregivers who are struggling with a loved one's severe autism a simple message: hang in there, keep breathing, and remember that feeling pain means that you are still alive. Pain reminds you that you are a living, breathing human and that's a beautiful feeling.

When it seems like nothing will get better with your loved one, you could spend your life focusing on the bad, but that will just make it all bad. The thing to do when you feel hopeless is find something good to take the place of the bad. Every day I wake up wishing for all my hopes and dreams; even if it seems like a long shot, that's what gets me through life.

It's also important to focus on what your child *can* do, rather than what they *can't*. If all you see are the challenges of autism, you will miss out on things that make your child great. Had I not had support and love from my family and friends, one of whom openly wept when he found out I wanted to end my life, my outlook on life would probably be different. I love life, and I always look forward to what comes around the corner. Always remember what you are fighting for and never give up. People care about you and love you even in darkness.

Mom:

Blake, this is a very good reflection of your feelings on this difficult subject. I wish it were simply "black and white," but this is complex.

The reading I have been doing recently by parents with severely autistic children is not so much about "the cure" but the utter exhaustion they face. So many parents would like to cure the harmful traits of autism, not get rid of their entire child. They are physically, mentally, socially and financially exhausted.

Imagine what it may be like to be a caregiver on duty 24/7 so that their child doesn't head bang; awaken many times throughout the night; have no time to relax or nurture other siblings; have little savings since money goes to therapies and respite workers; couples never being couples because they have to spell off each other to be with their child who is struggling to live in this perplexingly complicated world. These parents are often all alone because they've lost their old friends who just don't get their new reality.

Yes, these parents find joy and wonder in their child—seemingly small things like when he/she watches dust motes dance in the air, enjoys a new food, or when he/she is asleep and is so peacefully beautiful.

We can't begin to put ourselves in their shoes—the severely autistic child or his parents or siblings. It is an impossible world to truly know 100%. We can listen and support.

My thoughts for the day,

Mom

xoxo

Empathy and Learning to Be More Open-Minded

One big myth about autism is that we lack empathy. WRONG. Jami, my sister from another mother, reflected:

> Blake is compassionate, kind and an advocate for others. He has educated and helped others with autism throughout his life. He shares his story, helps people understand autism and has also inspired people like his parents to bring things forward in a political spotlight on a provincial and national level.

> One little boy by the name of Blake has made quite the impact for the autism spectrum...I wonder if he will ever know just how great that impact has been.

My mom told me there's a "double empathy problem." Basically, while it is true that autistic people may lack insight into non-autistic perceptions, it is equally the case that non-autistic people lack insight into the minds and culture of autistic people. So we autistics have gained a greater level of insight into non-autistic society, more than vice versa, probably because we have to in order to thrive in a non-autistic culture. Unless you have an autistic person in your life, you don't need to try to understand what makes us tick.

One of my dearest respite workers and family friends, Miranda, summarized what sounds like my philosophy of life:

> Blake may think and feel that he has been learning from all of us throughout his life, but I want him to know that he has been the one teaching us. Teaching us how to be patient, to enjoy the simple things—the value of family and our pets, to sit and watch cartoons every once in awhile to laugh, to be silly, to be brave, to say what's on our mind, to not be scared to try new things. He's taught us it's okay to be upset and then resolve it. Most of all, we've learned that when we have a passion and desire to do something to not stop until we've achieved it!

So yeah, I am different. Everyone is. Call me quirky, odd duck, whatever, I am me. I am proud. As my dad says, "Be a leader, not a follower." Although they may be biased, my parents said I am the most compassionate, caring, loving and empathetic person they know:

> Unprompted, Blake sends texts to people when they are feeling down, care packages to his gramps during COVID-19, housewarming gifts to former colleagues living across the country, thoughtful Christmas presents to neighbours of his cousins.
>
> He expresses concern and worry whenever a crisis occurs that may affect someone he knows. He lends money (he is learning not to!), but we all learn this lesson in our own time. He is bent on the belief that

everyone in society deserves a decent quality of life.
This is a tremendously valiant trait.

My autistic nature means that I think everyone should be treated
equally and fairly by government. This has raised an ongoing debate
with anyone who wants to listen to me. As I learn more, my thinking
is becoming more grey than black and white. On paper, communism
sounds utopian, but I am learning a more balanced set of political views.
Not all conservatives are evil, nor are all socialists perfect!

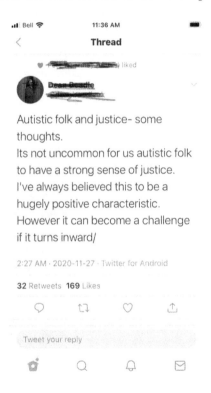

**Tweet capturing autistics' sense of justice,
black and white thinking**

No one is better equipped than close family friend John McAdam to
nudge me gradually to realize that the world's societies can be governed
by many different people and that it's good to keep an open mind. I
am learning to see that care, compassion and empathy for all aren't the
platforms of just one political party (that is, the left).

What follows was John's recall of one such conversation:

Blake and I sparred on the topic of politics. He was taking shots at conservative politics or alternately praising socialists and the virtues of communist politics. My initial approach was to deflect by saying that there are many views of politics and it can be a very personal matter. This didn't sit well with Blake who thought more in terms of black and white. Specifically, in Blake's mind, Stephen Harper, the Conservative Prime Minister of Canada at the time, was the devil incarnate who could not be drawn and quartered soon enough. Conservatives were lawless, irresponsible people who thought only of themselves. A patient explanation of the benefits of fiscal conservativism had all the traction of bedroom slippers on an ice rink.

So, feeling a little bit like the *Monty Python* character on the bridge with no arms and no legs but still game for the battle, I pulled out my last weapon with my teeth.

"Some think Stephen Harper is on the autism spectrum," I blurted out.

"What?" said Blake as he watched the horns on the devil incarnate fall off.

"It's true," I said.

Suddenly we were back on my ground talking about conservatives. I don't agree with everything Stephen Harper did, and his tone was less than compassionate, but he worked hard to create a favourable business climate in Canada which is an imperative of any modern nation where that wealth can be used for social good. Blake was interested in this new information, but even without horns, Harper was still the devil. I tried the approach of asking Blake to name one good thing about Stephen Harper. Evidently, there was no such thing.

So I asked Blake about something particularly egregious that Harper had done. Blake said he had cut funding for First Nations. I said I knew for a fact that First Nations funding was not cut to zero, so how much was cut? Well, Blake did not have a specific amount or know exactly what was cut.

"Blake," I said, "I have no clue either so isn't it a bit ridiculous that you and I are having a debate and neither one of us has a clue what the facts are?"

Blake thought about it for a bit and he agreed. WAHOOOOOO! The Deliverer of Unsolicited Advice finally scored a point...half a point maybe?

Recently, Blake received some very nice accolades from his workplace regarding his enthusiasm and thoroughness in covering local news. I certainly don't want to steal any of Blake's thunder, but maybe—just maybe—our discussion about facts and doing research contributed in some tiny way to the great job he is doing now. Also, he may be more open to considering the position of the "other side" in a debate because of our chats.

I have always had a great relationship with John, who I look up to as a fun "uncle." It wasn't until I turned eighteen that he started to talk to me like a father and give me life advice. John really helped me to look at conservatives in a different way and helped me understand that not all of them are greedy, aggressive billionaires like Donald Trump. I learned that many conservatives are good; Arnold Schwarzenegger comes to mind. I have learned I can't judge people before I get to know them. Politically, I consider myself a Left Libertarian who believes in individual choice and social equality. I vote for the person best suited to be a leader, switching between Liberal and NDP. I am blessed to have the McAdams in my life because they broaden my thinking and are always there for me.

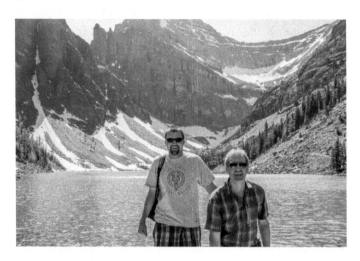

One of a *million* hikes with the McAdams. John and me taking a breather, Alberta *(courtesy L. McAdam)*

How It Feels to Have Autism

I was diagnosed with autism in kindergarten, but before that, my parents, family and friends knew I was different, as did I. I wasn't told I had autism until I was about nine years old, but once it was revealed, things in my life that I had questions about started to make sense. I did certain things no one else did, and I knew some of these things weren't "normal," but I did them anyway.

Marching Unencumbered to the Beat of My Own Drum

Apparently, I "march to the beat of my own drum." I am not influenced by fashion fads or peer popularity contests, nor do I care what people think when I do things that are different than the status quo. Is it because I am blind to others' perspectives or because I don't give a rat's ass? Maybe a bit of both.

One of my media mentors, Roz, said, "I remember Blake doing some Zumba at the recreation complex. He was right up there front and centre, encouraging others, especially kids, to come forward...it made people laugh, but in a good way. He was so obviously enjoying himself."

My mom said my cousin told her about the time I got up and danced on a mostly empty dance floor in downtown Montreal. I was literally dancing to my own beat and my cousin had never seen such uninhibited behaviour.

My sister from another mother, Sara, says she admired that I am following my true heart's desires and am not affected by the fear and judgment that often holds others back. It's a sentiment that Rebecca, my family friend, believes as well:

> Blake has been an inspiration to me in the ways of staying true to oneself and never caring what others think—because, frankly, why should we?! Before I met Blake, I was told he had autism, which made me think I had to act differently around him. But quickly after I met Blake, I realized that his open heart and his no-shame/no-judgment vibe allowed me to finally be free from all the ties I and others have placed on me. I felt free to express myself the way I wanted to and not to hide inside myself.
>
> Being around Blake continuously freed me from my cage. I thank Blake for that.

Her sister, Rachel, echoed this theme, "I have always admired Blake. I strive to be more like him: dancing in public, laughing out loud, jumping into the lake, challenging myself to let down my guard, being authentic, connecting with good people, saying exactly how I feel, being led by my heart."

Kristen, my lifelong family friend and job coach, remarked:

> Blake has a different kind of independence than most and it is hard to describe. But when he has come to

visit, I have been impressed with his desire to go off and do things on his own. He doesn't need someone else to accompany him to do the things he wants to do. Many people are afraid to do activities or explore a new city on their own, but it doesn't faze Blake. That's an admirable trait.

As you know, I spoke mostly through echolalia and repeated just about everything I heard when I was young. Sometimes I repeated things I heard on the radio, TV or a computer game, or I just talked to myself as a form of stimming along with flapping my arms and hands. My parents discouraged these behaviours in public for a long time because they felt they weren't socially appropriate even though they helped me cope with the complexity of the overwhelming world we live in. I knew they meant well by not allowing these stims in public because they wanted me to appear "normal" so that people would like me. They wanted me to be successful in life and knew that not many people at the time were accepting of unusual traits like stimming. I remember one time Mom was so frustrated when I was talking out loud to myself that she started whistling non-stop, I guess as a way of getting my attention. I was really hurt by this because I wasn't doing it on purpose to annoy her, it was just me stimming.

One of the most insightful, thoughtful family friends we have is Marie T. She described how it was getting to know me and how she simply saw me as me:

> I really got to start my own relationship with Blake when he was in the intermediate grades. I had never knowingly met anyone who was on the autism spectrum, so I didn't know what to expect. I met an intelligent, talented, interesting and sensitive young man. He may have repeated movie lines, but they were always the funny lines. He might have seemed a bit standoffish sometimes, but he did great job acting in local theatre. He may have repeated some stories, but geez, he sure knows a lot about a lot of things, including a lot about nature.

He is well-travelled and can make you feel like you are there when he shares his travel diaries. I have a photo of Blake, me and his mom after a boat cruise around Kingston. Blake has his arm around my shoulders but does not touch them. I do not see the sensory concern when I look at that photo. I see me having an excellent day with two friends.

Making eye contact is still difficult. I can do it much better than I used to because I almost never made eye contact with the people I talked to. Mom and Dad tried to teach me that making eye contact was important so that people knew I was listening to them. I didn't get it. What does eye contact have to do with listening? I was really frustrated when Mom or Dad would prompt me to make eye contact by saying, "Who are you talking to?" because it seemed like all they cared about was me making eye contact as opposed to caring about what I had to say. Forcing people to make eye contact is wrong, especially if it makes them feel uncomfortable. In fact, there are cultures out there that view eye contact, no pun intended, differently and think it's rude. So, if you wouldn't force a person from another culture that thinks eye contact is rude to make eye contact, why do it to an autistic person?

I am not mad at my parents for what they did in the past and the mistakes that they made (OCD kicking in here). They have done a wonderful job raising me and making me the person I am now. Kids don't come with instructions, and sometimes even the best parents in the world do things wrong. My parents were learning too! I just can't thank them enough for everything they have done. At the time, my parents just didn't understand that I was doing all of these things for a reason. They meant well.

Mr. Diebel, a.k.a. Mr. D, said some pretty nice things about my parents and me:

Blake has simply made his school and community better places to live. Awareness is the key to unlocking ignorance, and Blake has stood up proud of who he is and has made many others more in tune to the challenges faced by an individual on the autism spectrum.

When you meet Blake, you see a young man who is 6'5", handsome, well-dressed and has mature manners. This did not simply happen by osmosis. I have had the opportunity to review his entire educational experience through contact with his parents, previous school and school records, so I know him and his background well.

I have worked with students with challenging needs for over thirty years, and Blake is truly the poster boy of how a young man with many needs can overcome them with support. The most important pillar in this support is Blake himself. He truly appreciates the assistance he receives and leans on each other pillar when needed.

His home support is also paramount in that his parents, Jo and Ted, have been the foundation that has allowed Blake to grow into the young man he is. While Blake is a BIG Teddy bear, his autism challenges resulted in his parents spending countless hours becoming experts in the field which in turn helped Blake and the school system.

If I was diagnosed with autism as a child today, my parents probably would not have prevented me from stimming or forced me to make eye contact because more people have a better understanding of autism than they did in the nineties. They understand that hand flapping is how some people on the spectrum cope and making eye contact makes them uncomfortable. Even progressive employers understand this and they don't judge people on the spectrum when they stim. My guess is there are still lots of autistics who don't get past the job interview stage because their lack of eye contact is misinterpreted. This is one reason it is a good idea to disclose your autism and then emphasize your skills! It makes me feel good that attitudes are changing and we have a better understanding and acceptance of autism, something I wish we'd had when I was a kid.

I have autism but it doesn't have me. There are still things I struggle with, but everyone has challenges. One of my biggest issues is living with OCD and anxiety. I also still struggle to understand certain words and phrases as well as making direct eye contact. I am not cured (and I don't want to be), but I have overcome many things I used to struggle with like overstimulation, changes in routine and handling interpersonal conflict.

When I was in my early twenties, Kristen provided me with professional vocational advice. We had a huge argument where I verbally lashed out. While it was very distressing for both of us, I learned from this experience and now can better control my anger when disagreeing. Here's what she remembered:

> The conversation blew up and there was a lot of anger so we removed ourselves from the situation to give both of us time to process and calm down. After a chat with his parents and taking some space, Blake called me and apologized and we were able to keep working on things. When I think back to the times Blake had a difficult time coping, I was always impressed by his ability to pull back, take the time needed to process the situation and find a remedy he was comfortable with.

> In every situation of conflict, Blake makes amends with the person despite how heated a situation may have gotten. He has a humility in his interaction that is something we can all learn from. I always liked that Blake made the effort to talk to all people involved in a situation and get their perspective on why someone was thinking the way they were. I can't ever think of a time Blake didn't make things right and apologize.

Sometimes I was unsure of myself and my diagnosis of autism, and maybe I was somewhat prejudiced of my own disability. In college, I was reluctant to join an autism social group because the members didn't like to party or drink and were instead interested in seeing animated movies and other activities I wasn't interested in. I didn't realize I was being prejudiced because I just thought that I wasn't interested in joining the group. In reality, I didn't join because I only wanted to hang out with "normal" people. This was a mistake and it was no way to think, but I was still trying to figure out who I was. I wanted to try to be social outside of autism social groups. If I could turn back the clock, I would join this group. I would talk to the organizers about allowing people without autism to join so people on the spectrum could hang out with and meet other people without autism. Autistic people deserve to be included in society and in other social groups, not just ones that are organized exclusively for autistics.

That's another thing autistic people don't deserve—to be segregated just because we are different. It still bothers me that autistic children are sent to special schools instead of being in a regular public school. We may have challenges, but we are still human beings. Don't cut us off from the rest of the world!

Sadly, no matter where I go there will always be people who are either ignorant of autism or hate or fear people on the spectrum. Whenever I hear a tragic story involving autism, I just ignore it. Instead, I focus on the people in the world who are helping people like me and are doing good things. When it comes to bullies, I ignore them, too, and I tell myself they are not worth getting upset over.

How Hard Is It to be Kind and Inclusive? Three Affecting Stories

A close family friend, Gary King, said it best, "All people are unique; someone should not pass judgement on or negatively stereotype any individual because they are perceived as different. Instead, we should take the time to understand others' needs and abilities, to be kind and respectful."

The following three stories affected my mom a lot. The first two stories point out how my community responded to me—one poorly and the other positively. The third story touched us both and showed that we are not alone.

Story One: Ignoramus in Public Places (as told by my mom)

I used to be that person.

You know, the snotty woman in the checkout line who eye-rolled at misbehaving kids. *If only that parent would discipline their kid. If it was mine, I'd make him smarten up and quit whining.*

Ha!

Now I stick up for and quietly support that adult bearing witness to a meltdown—whether that child has autism or not.

After all, who am I to judge?

A new rubber ball for Blake! You know, the kind with bright wide red and blue stripes. His fingers tightly wrapped around the long-awaited toy. Spring is finally here. Time to bounce and catch a ball! I always seem to pick the wrong checkout lineup. It's only two-deep, but there's a bazillion items in the older guy's basket in front of us.

Blake is so patient, unlike me, his new ball gripped tightly in his hand. He could stand in line all day. He's entranced with his new ball and oblivious to the florescent lights flickering, loudspeaker crackling for a price check.

I turn my back for a split-second and glance at the fresh spring flower display. *Maybe I should treat myself? Oh, that would mean losing our spot and I can't leave Blake alone.* While pondering this impulse purchase, Blake lets out an ear-piercing scream and falls back into me.

What the hell just happened?! I only had my eyes off him for ten seconds...

"Get a grip, kid," the older guy yells. "What's wrong with you?"

The older guy and the cashier cluck, eye-roll and disparagingly agree that this is a spoilt brat with a lousy mother.

With lightning speed I go through the ABCs to ascertain what just occurred:

A = Antecedent, B = Behaviour, C = Consequence. Always a teachable moment for everyone involved.

A – Blake immersed with his new ball, unaware of others around him. I believe the older guy grabbed the ball out of Blake's hand to initiate a conversation.

B – Blake's outburst.

C – Older guy and cashier recoil.

Let's unpack this further. If Blake had been overtly disabled, let's say blind with a white cane or service dog, would that older guy have grabbed the ball from him to initiate conversation? I'm assuming he may have used his voice first, which would have elicited scaffolding conversation support from me in order for Blake to respond.

Anyway, there are too many public space horror stories to describe, but let's just say I use that time, when I have the mental energy, to educate and occasionally shame, I am ashamed to say.

If the crusty cashier from Canadian Tire is reading this, you know I'm talking about you.

Story Two: The Beauty of a Small Town

There are a million things we need to master as we grow toward independence. One of them is walking home from school. I needed to learn how to walk to my mom's office after school in Grade 4. The route was straightforward: exit the side door, cross the yard, use the crossing guard, cross the highway. Walk south for 1½ km on the sidewalk, crossing eight intersections (none busy and only one traffic light). I did a few practise runs with my mom following in the car. My incentive was a frozen yogurt cone.

My mom says this was a BIG day for me. She waited and watched through the storefront window for me to come hopping in. Well, it didn't quite go as planned. I got picked up by a family friend who insisted I get in—after all, I was autistic and it was unsafe to walk alone alongside a busy highway! My mom said she also got two phone calls from worried folks who saw me walking. "Has he run away?" "Is he okay?" Hey, I got my frozen yogurt faster than if I'd walked! The beauty of a small town! Next time I was told I had to walk and say a polite "No thank you" to any pickup offers if I wanted my cone.

One of the best parts in our "village" is autism families. This last story depicts the first time I met my autistic friend Jakob and when our moms connected for life.

Story Three: "Would You Like Some Tea?" (as told by my mom)

Blond curls, bubbly expression—what a sweet wee girl of about three or four.

Oblivious to her pretend tea party invitation, Blake intently lines up the forks and knives in the Fisher Price kitchen.

Another anxiety-provoking Parent Preschool Resource Centre drop-in session.

So, I engage with the Shirley Temple lookalike.

"Look, Blake, she'd like you to have some tea. Here's a cup. Say, I'd like to have tea please."

Radio silence. Blank stare at a wall.

I drop back to the couch, swallow back my fear and fight back tears amidst incessant parent chatter that goes something like, "So, are you going to put Laila in French immersion? Did you sign up Justin for hockey? What are you getting for Brendan's birthday party?"

In my head I think, *Do we have to send Blake away to southern Ontario to a special learning disabilities residential school? Are you kidding—French immersion? I'm hoping for a few English words someday. What birthday party?*

Beside the Fisher Price pretend kitchen, in the quiet corner of the centre are two easels and one rather kinetically active, dark-haired preschooler working on making an artistic mess of the primary colour paints as he wields his fat brush like a sword.

Taking Blake's hand, I guide him to the second easel. After a brief struggle adjusting to the plastic apron (sensory aversion!), he begins his masterpiece. At a glance, it looks like two typical boys having fun. It doesn't last long. But it was beautiful.

The best part was the boy's mom quietly approached me and said her boy wasn't talking much yet either. Maybe we could connect and have a play date sometime. My heart melted. My journey is no longer solo. Autism moms and autistic friends for life.

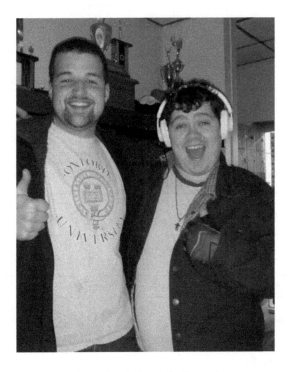

Buddies for life, Jakob and me

It Takes a Village: Underrated Heroes

It's a cliché, but as shown in the previous chapters, it truly *takes a village to raise a child.* I've lived, so far, in five different communities, and over the years I have made many friends and had so much support, both professionally and personally. Each has played a role in me becoming who I am today. Here's a sample of the numbers that make up my "village."

2 parents	10 EAs	10 autism families
3 grandparents	12 principals and VPs	100+ peers (school)
5 aunts and uncles	6 bus drivers	40 peers (college)
14 cousins	4 custodians	30 peers (workplace)
5 secondary family members	15 lunch/recess monitors	8 supervisors/bosses
4 neighbours	15 respite workers	17 roommates
6 babysitting family members	50+ family friends	4 day-care providers
48 teachers	2 life coaches	3 landlords
20 supply teachers	3 job coaches/developers	20 college professors
2 accessibility officers	5 social services navigators	2 family physicians
10 speech therapists	35 theatre mentors/peers	2 occupational therapists
1 physical therapist	3 psychologists	1 psychiatrist
1 nurse practitioner	15 service club supporters	50+ sports teammates

Speech Therapists

Speech-language pathologists (SLP) and communication disorders assistants (CDA) were the main supporters in my "village." SLPs and CDAs gave me and everyone who interacted with me the tools to learn how to communicate. I was lucky that my parents could afford to pay privately. I know my parents made financial sacrifices to make sure I had speech therapy, respite workers, social skills tutors, pre-vocational coaches and life coaches. There were no publicly available services after I aged out at six. I received one eight-week block and then no more. Do people think we magically aren't autistic anymore at age six?!

Extended Family

I am fortunate to have supportive family—lots of aunts, uncles and cousins. Uncle Randy, Aunt Helen, cousins Nick, Steven and Danielle showed their kindness here: "Blake has grown to be an amazing young man with a kind and thoughtful heart. Blake's given us the ability to understand and recognize autism in others. We are fortunate to have Blake in our family and appreciate his talents and gifts. He taught us to be patient, inclusive and grateful for the family we have."

Gramps Shares His Thoughts on Having an Autistic Grandson

Ah! Blake—The Beginning! Grandma Roseanne to the rescue. It was a cold eight-hour drive from London to Espanola in early February 1994. I was just a spectator—I am not good with babies! We would always be there to support Blake, Jo and Ted from day one.

As for his diagnosis and challenges, Grandma Roseanne and I never fretted about it. Growing up in the 1930-40s we had some peers that were "slower" in school, but it was no big deal; it just was the way it was. While we had concerns about what Blake's future would hold, we felt that natural worry for all our grandkids. Our role as grandparents did not change with Blake—we were proud of all his efforts and accomplishments, especially his educational achievements and his efforts at giving sports a go despite not being an all-star.

We could see that sometimes Blake acted a bit differently than his cousins—like pacing and self-talking. We learned that this is stimming and it helps him process his environment and control his feelings. You know, we all have unique strengths, weaknesses and traits. I tried hard to be more practical and keep the emotions out of it. Rather than focusing on what Blake couldn't do, I'd say, "Let him try." Blake's willingness to take on things is a great characteristic of his. He is not afraid. I'd support him even if he ran for prime minister!

Distance has played a big role in how often we got to see Blake and his parents. Living far away meant we weren't part of his day-to-day life, but frequent calls kept us abreast. We had faith in his parents working hard on his behalf to make sure he got what he needed to thrive. Having very supportive extended families, on both sides, allowed Blake to soar, leave home, go to college and live and work in different provinces knowing that when times are rough, he will always have family to fall back on. This makes him resilient and strong.

Tobacco Lake family camp memories will live on forever. Fishing, swimming, boating. Blake and I went fishing on many nights—just the two of us, which was good quiet time for us both! We never met a cast iron frying pan and fish fillets we didn't like!

Grandma Roseanne was his biggest cheerleader. I am so proud of Blake and love him dearly!

Gramps

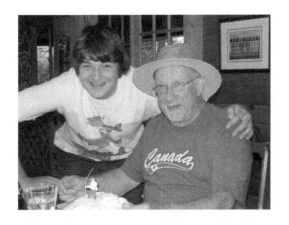

One of my fiercest supporters, my gramps!

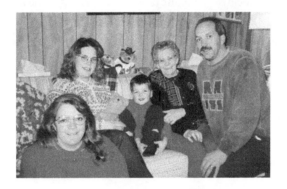

My Priddle clan

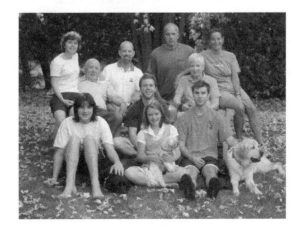

My Beyers clan

Family Friends

We have a ton of family friends scattered across Canada. Everyone has grown up around me and has accepted me for who I am while supporting me wherever I hang my hat. Eliza, a lifelong family friend, shared her reflections:

> I am so proud to call Blake my friend. He has done so well and conquered so many things that are scary enough for people not on the spectrum (i.e., college, moving away from home). I admire how brave he is about taking jobs so far away from home (Yellowknife, The Pas) because it means he follows his passion for radio. I look up to Blake in that sense, and I'm hoping that if the time comes where I need to move far away to follow a career I love I will be able to show the same bravery.

Respite Workers and Life Coaches

Unbeknownst to me, I had an impact on the career trajectory of my Grade 5-6 respite worker, Miranda:

> What an amazing man Blake has become. He has had the most amazing support team behind him (his parents). I was always very humbled and honoured to watch his amazing parents love, encourage and support him every day.
>
> I talk about Blake often: how proud I am of him, how brave he is, and how he has overcome so many obstacles to become who he is. He has shown me my passion in life, which is to help others who are on the spectrum. I truly believe everything happens for a reason. We were meant to be in each other's lives for some time, after all he has taught me more about myself and the path my life needed to take. He has opened my eyes on special

needs and that everyone is different and accepted in their own way.

Blake and his family hold a very special part in my heart and mean a lot to me. I am honoured to have been part of his childhood.

Autism Families

It's easy to be in the company of autism families. We all "get it" because there's no need to explain our quirky behaviours. There is diversity within the autism spectrum and the human gene pool. Sure, we have social communication and sensory challenges, but we are all individuals. Vicky Miron, my respite worker and mom to my good friend Jakob, echoed this sentiment:

> I think we had a good time together. Blake taught us as much as we taught him, and we learned how different individuals could be with an ASD diagnosis. Blake and Jakob complemented each other and were as different as day and night.

> It was an honour to be part of Blake's achievements and watch him grow into a man. The small boy who wouldn't try anything became the man who flew out west and lives alone. Way to go Blake!

My Parents

These are their final thoughts:

> We dream of a day where there is no more "inspiration porn." You know, those social media clips where the Toronto Blue Jays all show up at an autistic boy's birthday party because his mom posted online that no one came to his party. Or the feel-good news clip that the local coffee shop hired some disabled adults.

Why?

Kids should naturally be invited to attend parties regardless of ability, race or creed. All people should have meaningful employment, and employers should hire all with some ability to contribute to a job without making a big to-do about it.

We realize inspiration is a double-edged sword. Blake wrote this book, in part, to inspire, to give hope and to show how personal and societal adversity can be tackled.

After all, with these shared stories, awareness and understanding grows, leading to inclusion of diversity in all its stripes alongside banishing the word "normal" from our everyday vernacular.

In our dream, everyone is free to just be

Belong and thrive

Regardless of race, age, ability, gender expression, geographic location,

To reach their own potential.

You've Been Listening to Your Host, Blake "Crash" Priddle

My life with autism has been mostly wonderful, and I would never trade it for anything. I would gladly trade my OCD and anxiety for a cold beer any day, but I don't have that option. I am lucky to have a family that supports me every step of the way, and friends and work colleagues to help as well. Sadly, some people on the spectrum aren't as lucky and are put down, excluded and bullied for being different. Many in our society still don't know enough about autism to understand how a person on the spectrum is feeling or how they do things. Worst of all, autistic children and adults don't receive the services they need in many places because they aren't available or because governments make funding cuts.

Things are better than they were back when I was diagnosed in the late nineties, but we can do better. I am really impressed with how the overall environment has recently improved for autistic people. A lot of things we have now would have been beneficial for me growing up—like movie theatres that offer sensory friendly screenings and some places that allow autistic children to fast track line-ups. It is increasingly common for autistics to wear headphones in noisy environments, and stimming is becoming more and more acceptable. Today when people expect me to look at them, I just say I am sorry but I don't like making direct eye contact and that it has nothing to do with them, it just makes me feel uncomfortable.

The next time you see someone out in public doing something unusual that you think is weird or wrong, don't assume they are misbehaving or that their parents aren't taking action; it may be autism related. If you are an employer and are interviewing someone who is not making eye contact or misreads a social cue, don't assume it's because they don't care or they're not listening; they may be autistic. Stimming and Parkinson's movements are uncontrollable. You wouldn't tell a person with Parkinson's to stop shaking, so why make an autistic person stop stimming? If a person with autism needs a sensory break from over-stimulation, it's no different than a person with diabetes taking time out to have some juice.

Martin Luther King Jr. had a dream that one day his children would live in a nation where they aren't judged by the colour of their skin. I have a dream that one day we will live in a nation—no, a world—where everyone with autism is accepted for who they are and not judged. I dream of a world where money and greed doesn't get in the way of providing services for autistic people to help them live their dreams. Society has made mistakes in the way it treats those who are "different," but we have the power to change the future and embrace new inclusive schools, workplaces and communities.

I hope you enjoyed reading *Good Morning, Blake*—my journey so far!

This is Blake "Crash" Priddle signing off for now. I grew up autistic and I'm more than okay.

Afterword

Removing the Bubble Wrap

My parents, after consulting with me about content, presented at a national Worktopia Connects Conference in 2018. They were asked a number of questions that related to the themes of the conference: "Exploring the Transition to Adulthood for a Young Adult with ASD and the Impact It Has on the Role of the Family Supporting Them Towards Independence."

They called their presentation "Removing the Bubble Wrap."[8] What follows is an excerpt:

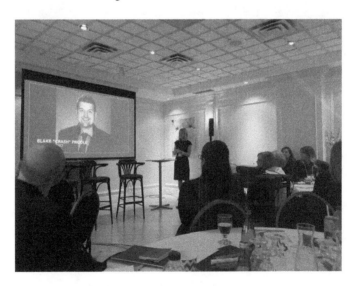

Screengrab taken at Worktopia

---

[8] "Removing the Bubble Wrap" implies taking a person out of their comfort zone with the aim of getting them to learn, grow and thrive to the best of their potential.

How would you describe the experience of having an autistic son transition to adulthood?

In a word: ROLLER COASTER.

Parenting in general is like being on a roller coaster.

Parenting a kid with ASD is like being on a roller coaster in the DARK!

What words of advice would you give parents whose children are approaching transition age?

- If you choose to "remove the bubble wrap," be ready for hard work, frustration, exhaustion, meltdowns, suicidal ideation… and incredible moments of beaming proudness beyond compare!
- It's OK to fall apart periodically (Jo took two "timeouts" in two decades to get herself mentally healthy).
- Focus on your kid's strengths.
- Listen to your kid and what their passions are. Your job is to help clear the path.
- Make your kid get a job by the time he/she is fifteen. According to Temple Grandin (and Blake) this is mega-important. Blake learned so much in the three years he cleaned bathrooms, mopped floors, pushed carts in -20°C weather, dealt with rude customers…
  - Time management (was never late or missed a shift in three years)
  - Financial management (opened his first bank account, learned when you spend there's no more)
  - Some tasks suck (all jobs—even your dream job—has stuff you don't like doing)
  - Responsibility and being loyal to the company
  - Flexible thinking (after two years, Blake agreed to have his name on the on-call list for extra shifts).
- We are in it for the long haul as parents. We need to be lifelong advocates to ensure our society is as inclusive as possible. It might mean organizing a protest, signing a petition, having lunch with your MP/MPP/MLA.

- Be prepared to be lifelong navigators of sectors and systems that change like the wind and don't make sense...be it mental-health care, employment services, respite providers, financial planning, housing options...
- Surround your kid with an army of allies to help champion what he deserves.
- Go with your gut. You as parents are the experts (besides your kid, of course!).
- Focus on one step at a time. Thinking too far ahead can be anxiety-provoking.
- Lastly, and most importantly, believe in your kid.

When we *removed the bubble wrap*, Blake failed lots. There were (and always will be, actually) lots of bumps and bruises. We are under no illusions—more will happen. THAT'S LIFE!

Jo Beyers (Mom) and Ted Priddle (Dad)

Acknowledgements

This book took a lot of hard work over three years to complete. I couldn't have done it without the contributions from my friends and family who took the time to help me write my story.

I thank everyone in my life who helped me to overcome every single obstacle and to those who are still in my corner helping me to this day.

Thanks to all the school and college staff and peers who were willing to go out of their way to help me succeed.

A big shout out to my employers, past and present, for giving me a chance and making the workplace inclusive. And to fellow employees who support me and give me constructive feedback as I continue to get better at my craft.

I thank my mother and father for raising me into the man I have become.

Thumbs up to Lanny Bowley and Jeannine Rosenberg for making this book readable, and to the talented Tellwell Publishing team for bringing it to life.

Special thanks to Dr. Temple Grandin for granting permission to cite an excerpt of her interview with me, use her photo, and for providing a book cover blurb.

Kudos to those who provided blurbs for the book to help draw attention to potential readers in the autism community and beyond.

I want to thank you, the reader, for purchasing my book and taking time to read my story. I hope you learned something new and feel hope.

Last but not least, I would like to thank my beloved Grandma Roseanne for the contribution she made for the book, and for always believing in me and encouraging me to live life to its fullest. Sadly, she passed away before the book was completed.

My story is still going on as we speak. Follow my journey on my Facebook page and my website https://www.blakecrashpriddle.com/.

Blake "Crash" Priddle

Citations

Introduction:
Grandin, T. *Different...Not Less: Inspiring Stories of Achievement and Successful Employment from Adults with Autism, Asperger's, and ADHD*. Arlington, TX: Future Horizons; 2012.

Chapter 1:
Dr. Stephen Shore is an autism expert who served as the keynote speaker for Lime Connect's annual *Leading Perspectives on Disability* reception on March 22, 2018, in New York City.

https://www.limeconnect.com/opportunities_news/detail/leading-perspectives-on-disability-a-qa-with-dr-stephen-shore

Gentles, S. J., Nicholas, D. B., Jack, S. M., McKibbon, K. A., & Szatmari, P. (2019). Coming to understand the child has autism: A process illustrating parents' evolving readiness for engaging in care. *Autism*, 1-14. Doi:10.1177/1362361319874647

Chapter 2:
Cited with permission from author's publisher: Matthews, Andrew. (1990). *Making Friends: A Guide to Getting Along With People*. (p. 129). Singapore: Media Masters.

See https://seashell.com.au/ for complete list of resources by Andrew Matthews.

Chapter 3:
Dennis Debbaudt's autism and law enforcement content and curriculum development has set the standard for autism training for policing, public safety and criminal justice professionals in the US, Canada and globally. https://autismriskmanagement.com/

Chapter 5:

Beyers, J., & Di Ruggiero, E. (Oct. 2018). *Hiding in Plain View...How Socially Accountable are We for Those with Invisible Dis/Abilities?* The Global Community Engaged Medical Education Muster Conference, Mt Gambier, Australia.

Afterword:

Worktopia is a national employment network with a shared goal to change the odds of employment success for people on the autism spectrum. https://worktopia.ca/